THE LEARNING HEALTH SYS

VALUING AMERICA'S HEALTH

Aligning Financing to Reward Better Health and Well-Being

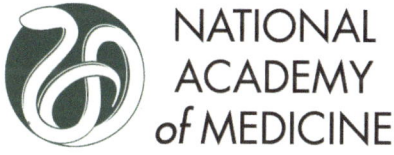

WASHINGTON, DC
NAM.EDU

THE NATIONAL ACADEMIES PRESS
Washington, DC
www.nap.edu

NATIONAL ACADEMY OF MEDICINE   500 Fifth Street, NW   Washington, DC 20001

This publication has undergone peer review according to procedures established by the National Academy of Medicine (NAM). Publication by the NAM signifies that it is the product of a carefully considered process and is a contribution worthy of public attention but does not constitute endorsement of conclusions and recommendations by the NAM. The views presented in this publication are those of individual contributors and do not represent formal consensus positions of the authors' organizations; the NAM; or the National Academies of Sciences, Engineering, and Medicine.

This initiative was convened with support from the George Family Foundation, Nemours, Samueli Foundation, Well Being Trust, and Whole Health Institute. Any opinions, findings, or conclusions expressed in this publication do not necessarily reflect the views of any organization or agency that assisted in the development of this project.

International Standard Book Number-13: 978-0-309-70620-9
International Standard Book Number-10: 0-309-70620-3
Digital Object Identifier: https://doi.org/10.17226/27141
Library of Congress Control Number: 2023948064

Copyright 2024 by the National Academy of Sciences. All rights reserved.

Printed in the United States of America.

Suggested citation: National Academy of Medicine. 2024. *Valuing America's Health: Aligning Financing to Reward Better Health and Well-Being*. Hm. Pham, M. Chesney, D. Chisolm, D. Erickson, C. Koller, P. Long, L. G. Moore, L. M. Nichols, A. Offodile, C. Powell, J. Sharfstein, D. Shurney, S. Szanton, J. Lee, J. L. Flaubert, M. Cocchiola, P. S. Chua, A. Anise, and A. Hunt, *editors*. NAM Special Publication. Washington, DC: The National Academies Press.

*"Knowing is not enough; we must apply.
Willing is not enough; we must do"*
—GOETHE

LEADERSHIP
INNOVATION
IMPACT

for a healthier future

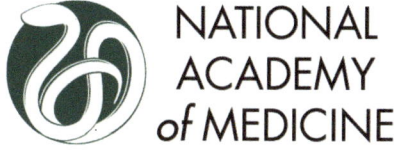

NATIONAL
ACADEMY
of MEDICINE

ABOUT THE NATIONAL ACADEMY OF MEDICINE

The **National Academy of Medicine** is one of three Academies constituting the National Academies of Sciences, Engineering, and Medicine (the National Academies). The National Academies provide independent, objective analysis and advice to the nation and conduct other activities to solve complex problems and inform public policy decisions. The National Academies also encourage education and research, recognize outstanding contributions to knowledge, and increase public understanding in matters of science, engineering, and medicine.

The **National Academy of Sciences** was established in 1863 by an Act of Congress, signed by President Lincoln, as a private, nongovernmental institution to advise the nation on issues related to science and technology. Members are elected by their peers for outstanding contributions to research. Dr. Marcia McNutt is president.

The **National Academy of Engineering** was established in 1964 under the charter of the National Academy of Sciences to bring the practices of engineering to advising the nation. Members are elected by their peers for extraordinary contributions to engineering. Dr. John L. Anderson is president.

The **National Academy of Medicine** (formerly the Institute of Medicine) was established in 1970 under the charter of the National Academy of Sciences to advise the nation on issues of health, health care, and biomedical science and technology. Members are elected by their peers for distinguished contributions to medicine and health. Dr. Victor J. Dzau is president.

Learn more about the National Academy of Medicine at NAM.edu.

VALUING AMERICA'S HEALTH: ALIGNING FINANCING TO REWARD BETTER HEALTH AND WELL-BEING

Steering Group Members

HOANGMAI PHAM *(Chair)*, Institute for Exceptional Care
MARGARET CHESNEY, University of California, San Francisco
DEENA CHISOLM, Nationwide Children's Hospital
DAVID ERICKSON, Federal Reserve Bank of New York
CHRISTOPHER KOLLER, Milbank Memorial Fund
PETER LONG, Blue Shield of California
L. GORDON MOORE, Goodside Health
LEN M. NICHOLS, The Urban Institute
ANAEZE OFFODILE, MD Anderson Cancer Center
CHERYL POWELL, Ad Hoc LLC
JOSHUA SHARFSTEIN, Johns Hopkins University
DEXTER SHURNEY, Adventist Health
SARAH SZANTON, Johns Hopkins University

NAM Staff

Development of this publication was facilitated by contributions of the following NAM staff, under the guidance of J. Michael McGinnis, Leonard D. Schaeffer Executive Officer and Executive Director of the NAM Leadership Consortium:

JENNIFER LEE, Visiting Scholar *(until April 2022)*
JENNIFER LALITHA FLAUBERT, Program Officer
MICHAEL COCCHIOLA, Associate Program Officer *(until July 2022)*
PEAK SEN CHUA, Consultant
AMANDA HUNT, Senior Program Officer *(from August 2022)*
AYODOLA ANISE, Deputy Director, NAM Leadership Consortium *(until February 2023)*
SHARYL NASS, Director of the Board on Health Care Services
JENNA L. OGILVIE, Deputy Director of Communications *(until April 2023)*
MADELEINE DEYE, Editorial Projects Coordinator
TOCHI OGBU-MBADIUGHA, Senior Program Assistant *(until June 2022)*

DISCLOSURE OF CONFLICTS OF INTEREST

L. GORDON MOORE discloses former employment by 3M Information Systems.

JOSHUA SHARFSTEIN discloses personal fees from Sachs Policy Group, a health care and health care payment consulting company.

NAM LEADERSHIP CONSORTIUM
Collaboration for a Learning Health System

MARK B. McCLELLAN (*Chair*), Duke University
AMY ABERNETHY, Verily
SHANTANU AGRAWAL, Anthem Inc.
JEFFREY BALSER, Vanderbilt University Medical Center
GEORGES BENJAMIN, American Public Health Association
RACHELE BERRIA, AstraZeneca
DAVID BLUMENTHAL, The Commonwealth Fund
NAKELA COOK, PCORI
KAREN DeSALVO, Google
JUDITH FAULKNER, Epic Systems
DAVID FEINBERG, Cerner
JULIE L. GERBERDING, Merck & Co., Inc.
SANDRA HERNANDEZ, California Health Care Foundation
DIANE HOLDER, UPMC Health Plan
MICHELE HOOD, American Hospital Association
FREDERICK ISASI, Families USA
ADAM LENKOWSKY, Bristol Myers Squibb
PETER LONG, Blue Shield of California
JAMES L. MADARA, American Medical Association
LAURA MAURI, Medtronic
SUZANNE MIYAMOTO, American Academy of Nursing
VALERIE MONTGOMERY RICE, Morehouse School of Medicine
MARY D. NAYLOR, University of Pennsylvania
HAROLD PAZ, Stony Brook University
JONATHAN B. PERLIN, The Joint Commission
RICHARD PLATT, Harvard Medical School
DWAYNE PROCTOR, Missouri Foundation for Health
KYU RHEE, CVS Health, Aetna
LEWIS G. SANDY, UnitedHealth Group
LEONARD D. SCHAEFFER, University of Southern California
BRUCE SIEGEL, America's Essential Hospitals
DAVID SKORTON, Association of American Medical Colleges
JENNIFER TAUBERT, Johnson & Johnson
REED V. TUCKSON, Tuckson Health
DEBRA B. WHITMAN, AARP

NAM Leadership Consortium Staff

LAURA ADAMS, Senior Counsel
AYODOLA ANISE, Deputy Director (*until February 2023*)
SARAH GREENE, Senior Counsel
AMANDA HUNT, Senior Program Officer
SUNITA KRISHNAN, Program Officer (*since December 2022*)
J. MICHAEL McGINNIS, Executive Director
ANNIE MURFF, Senior Program Assistant
STEPHANIE STAN, Research Associate (*since June 2023*)
ASIA WILLIAMS, Program Officer

ACKNOWLEDGMENTS

The Steering Group would like to thank members of the Health Financing Writing Group, who helped develop and provide independent feedback on the Special Publication's care financing and economics content featured in sections 4 and 5. The members of the group are as follows.

JI IM, Senior Director, Community and Population Health, Common Spirit
DAN POLSKY, Bloomberg Distinguished Professor of Health Policy and Economics, Johns Hopkins University
LAUREN TAYLOR, Assistant Professor, Langone School of Medicine, New York University

The Steering Group would also like to thank Maggie Super Church for her contributions in understanding the design, implementation, impact, and current developments related to the Healthy Neighborhoods Study along with the Healthy Neighborhood Equity Fund I and II. Maggie Super Church serves as an independent consultant and the former vice president for healthy and resilient communities at the Conservation Law Foundation.

REVIEWERS

This Special Publication was reviewed in draft form by the Steering Group, who were chosen for their diverse perspectives and technical expertise, in accordance with review procedures established by the National Academy of Medicine (NAM).

We wish to thank the following individuals for their contributions:

ALICE CHEN, Covered California
MARSHALL CHIN, University of Chicago
CHRIS DeMARS, Oregon Health Authority
CHRISTOPHER B. FORREST, Children's Hospital of Philadelphia
ROBERT GALVIN, Blackstone
NEAL HALFON, University of California, Los Angeles
RACHEL WERNER, University of Pennsylvania
CHARLENE WONG, North Carolina Department of Health and Human Services

The reviewers listed above provided many constructive comments and suggestions, but they were not asked to endorse the content of the publication and did not see the final draft before it was published. Review of this publication was overseen by **AYODOLA ANISE,** Deputy Director, Leadership Consortium; **PEAK SEN CHUA,** Consultant; **JENNIFER LALITHA FLAUBERT,** Program Officer; **AMANDA HUNT,** Senior Program Officer; and **J. MICHAEL McGINNIS,** Leonard D. Schaeffer Executive Officer. Responsibility for the final content of this publication rests entirely with the editors and the NAM.

CONTENTS

Preface xv

Acronyms and Abbreviations xvii

Introduction and Initiative Background 1

1 Valuing America's Health 7

2 A Vision for Better Health and Well-Being 17

3 Prioritizing Whole Person and Whole Population Health and Well-Being 35

4 Investment Goals and Priority Actions 77

5 Health Transformation Through Disruptive Change 119

APPENDIXES

A Financing That Rewards Better Health and Well-Being Workshop Series Participant Suggestions. 123
B Stakeholder-Specific Priority Actions by Impact and Feasibility. . . 127
C Illustrative Models of Implementing Whole Person, Whole Population Health Priority Actions 139

BOXES, FIGURES, AND TABLE

BOXES

1 Steering Group Members, 3
2 Key Pillars of the Vision for Whole Person and Whole Population Health and Well-Being, 18
3 Innovative Whole Person and Whole Population Health Service Providers, 80
4 Housing Stability: Aligning Federal Policies with the Vision for Whole Person, Whole Population Health, 140
5 Food Security: Aligning Federal Policies with the Vision for Whole Person, Whole Population Health, 144

FIGURES

1 Whole person health in the context of whole population health, 4
2 Life expectancy for OECD countries, 8
3 U.S. Veterans Health Administration Circle of Health, 40
4 Key components of multi-stakeholder community collaborations, 84
5 Sample dynamics of disruptive policy | housing stability, 139
6 Sample dynamics of disruptive policy | food security, 143

TABLE

1 Whole Health Service Use Among Veterans with Chronic Pain, Mental Health Diagnoses, and Chronic Conditions from the First Quarter of 2017 to the Third Quarter of 2019, 42

PREFACE

Whole person, whole population health—the ability for people and populations to thrive and attain their full, optimized potential for health and well-being—is the ultimate goal of a healthy nation. Unfortunately, the United States faces a crisis in our collective health and well-being: declining life expectancy driven by long-standing and deepening inequities, a global pandemic, and the persistent inefficiency, ineffectiveness, and high cost of the nation's health and health care system.

A response proportional to this crisis is required. To mobilize real-world implementation, the National Academy of Medicine (NAM) convened 13 eminent experts, with experience across care financing and payment, equity and community engagement, and private capital markets, to review a full set of opportunities, levers, and disruptive forces that could uproot dominant fee-for-service interests and effect a shift toward whole person, whole population health.

This NAM Special Publication, *Valuing America's Health: Aligning Financing to Reward Better Health and Well-Being*, clearly underscores the urgency for the nation to reckon with the glaring shortfalls in the nation's health system. It also describes why health cannot be financed, delivered, and sustained by the health and health care sector alone. Health consequences are resident in virtually every decision, policy, and action taken throughout the individuals, organizations, and sectors that constitute our nation's society and economy. Furthermore, with the necessary leadership from government, and grassroots demand for solutions from communities, all members of society can contribute to an immediate, forceful, and momentous shifting of values, incentives, and culture that are both exogenous and endogenous to the health and health care system. Finally, the Special Publication outlines transformative actions that will help critical system stakeholders to more effectively execute responsibilities for our collective health and well-being.

The partnership between the NAM and the involved stakeholders is part of extensive and ongoing contributions to transformative health financing. Over the past 2 years, the NAM has conducted a phased release of nine sectoral impact assessments and an associated discussion of cross-cutting policy implications. The final synthesis publication was released in August 2022. In 2021, the NAM conducted a broad appraisal of the Center for Medicare & Medicaid Innovation (CMMI) on the effectiveness of alternative payment models, gaps in data collection to support equity, and opportunities to engage beneficiaries, businesses, payers, and providers more meaningfully. The resultant publication, the *CMMI Opportunity Agenda*, was released in September 2022 and has already informed CMMI's current strategic plan.

Given these contributions, it is clear that additional partnerships, cross-sectoral connections, and continuous engagement are required to realize this Special Publication's vision of whole person, whole population health. We look forward to assisting in the achievement of that vision.

J. Michael McGinnis, MD, MPP
Leonard D. Schaeffer Executive Officer
National Academy of Medicine

Hoangmai Pham, MD, MPH
President
Institute for Exceptional Care

ACRONYMS AND ABBREVIATIONS

ACA	Affordable Care Act
ACAP	Association for Community Affiliated Plans
ACO	accountable care organization
ASTHO	Association of State and Territorial Health Officials
BIPOC	Black, Indigenous, and People of Color
CAPABLE	Community Aging in Place: Advancing Better Living for Elders
CAPGI	Collaborative Approach to Public Good Investments
CBO	community-based organization
CDFI	Community Development Financial Institution
CHA	Community Health Assessment
CHART	Community Health Access and Rural Transformation
CHIP	Children's Health Insurance Program
CHIP	community health improvement plan
CHNA	community health needs assessment
CLF	Conservation Law Foundation
CMMI	Center for Medicare & Medicaid Innovation
CMS	Centers for Medicare & Medicaid Services
COVID-19	coronavirus disease 2019
D-SNP	Dual Eligible Special Needs Plan
EHR	electronic health record
EIA	environmental impact assessment
EPSDT	Early and Periodic Screening, Diagnostic, and Treatment
ERISA	Employee Retirement Income Security Act of 1974
ESG	Environmental, Social, and Governance

FIDE-SNP	Fully Integrated Dual Eligible Special Needs Plan
FMAP	Federal Medical Assistance Percentage
FQHC	Federally Qualified Health Center
FY	fiscal year
GDP	gross domestic product
HCBS	home- and community-based services
HEDIS	Healthcare Effectiveness Data and Information Set
HHS	U.S. Department of Health and Human Services
HIA	health impact assessment
HIDE-SNP	Highly Integrated Dual Eligible Special Needs Plan
HNEF	Healthy Neighborhood Equity Fund
HNS	Healthy Neighborhoods Study
HUD	U.S. Department of Housing and Urban Development
IRIS	Include, Respect, I Self-Direct
LISC	Local Initiatives Support Coalition
LTSS	long-term services and supports
MBE	Minority Business Enterprise
MedPAC	Medicare Payment Advisory Commission
MLR	medical loss ratio
MMA	Medicaid Modernization Act of 2003
NAM	National Academy of Medicine
NIMHD	National Institute on Minority Health and Health Disparities
NIST	National Institute of Standards and Technology
NOLA	New Orleans, Louisiana
OECD	Organisation for Economic Co-operation and Development
PACE	Program of All-Inclusive Care for the Elderly
PCMH	patient-centered medical home
PIB	Proceedings of a Workshop—in Brief
REIT	Real Estate Investment Trust
ROI	return on investment

SAS	Statistical Analysis System
SBHC	school-based health center
SCF	Southcentral Foundation
SDoH	social determinants of health
SIM	State Innovation Model
SNAP	Supplemental Nutritional Assistance Program
SNP	Special Needs Plan
VA	U.S. Department of Veterans Affairs
VBC	value-based care
VBP	value-based payment
VHA	Veterans Health Administration
WHS	Whole Health System of Care
WI DHS	Wisconsin Department of Health Services

INTRODUCTION AND INITIATIVE BACKGROUND

The COVID-19 pandemic has not affected all health institutions[1] equally. Some systems suffered financially when non-urgent visits and procedures were canceled or deferred. Meanwhile, advanced value-based payment models[2] remained financially resilient, launching innovative programs to support individuals and communities[3] as the pandemic was ongoing. The renewed interest in value-based payment models as a mechanism to deliver quality at lower prices and reduce dependence on care volumes prompted interest in examining the models of care that were effective in promoting whole person health, along with the payment structures needed to support them (Morse, 2020). In the spring of 2021, the National Academy of Medicine's (NAM's) Leadership Consortium, in collaboration with the Health and Medicine Division of the National Academies of Sciences, Engineering, and Medicine, held a 3-day workshop series titled Financing That Rewards Better Health and Well-Being (NASEM, 2021a).

The workshop brought together experts and leaders from health care delivery organizations, public health, payers, health services research, patients, and families to conceptualize a path forward for delivering equitable and high-quality care oriented to whole person and whole population health and well-being. The workshop focused on the need to transform the current model of U.S. health financing from its current framework, which rewards the volume of services

---

[1] Health institutions refer to organizations that provide health care and related services.
[2] Value-based payment (VBP), or value-based care (VBC), models hold physicians, clinicians, and care facilities accountable for quality and cost through shared financial risk. They often assume a pay-for-performance fashion by tying compensation to performance measures. Advanced VBP models include bundled payments, accountable care organizations (ACOs), and global capitation.
[3] Communities are places where people live, learn, work, and play. Community-driven solutions are led by community members to change local factors that can influence health and health equity, and, if successful, expand beyond a single locality. Community leaders can be regular citizens, local political leaders, or members of anchor institutions such as churches, hospitals, and schools.

provided, to a model that incentivizes payment approaches that are person-centered, integrative, and holistic in advancing individual, community, and population health. The objectives included:

- Identifying examples of policies, clinical/nonclinical strategies, and payment models that are focused on patient outcomes and advancing health equity;
- Considering barriers and opportunities to scaling innovative payment models and approaches; and
- Discussing strategies for transforming health financing to improve equity and individual and population health.

A Proceedings of a Workshop—in Brief (PIB), which highlighted presentations and discussions from the workshop was published in September 2021 (NASEM, 2021a). Important themes from the workshop as well as proposed implementation actions from the PIB are briefly summarized in Appendix A (NASEM, 2021a). Following the conclusion of the workshop, the Workshop Planning Committee transitioned to a Steering Group that has met regularly to develop this Special Publication (see Box 1). The Steering Group identified approaches to elaborate on the workshop themes; and posed and identified a unified vision, measurable goals, and specific action steps that various stakeholders can use to transform health delivery and payment systems to produce more equitable health and well-being at the individual, community, and population levels. The Steering Group also established a subgroup focused specifically on supplemental financing and funding strategies (as opposed to care payment approaches) to improve whole person and whole population health. This subgroup assisted the Steering Group in developing the insights laid out in this Special Publication, adding context on ways to leverage and catalyze non-conventional sources of capital for investments in whole person and whole population health. Finally, the report engaged stakeholders such as Maggie Super Church to better understand the elements of healthy neighborhoods, such as access to food, affordable housing, available public transport, and high-quality education.

This Special Publication elaborates on the themes addressed in the workshop and looks beyond whole health care models to identify society-level interventions that can be used to maintain and promote equitable health and well-being. From the vantage point of health care and public health experts, this Special Publication also explores measurable goals and identifies several levers, mechanisms, and policies that various stakeholders can take to advance individual and community health. However, these opportunities for action are not meant to be exhaustive or prescriptive; systems across states, localities, and stakeholders vary too much to provide this guidance. Additionally, the publication does not detail payment

> **BOX 1**
>
> *Steering Group Members*
>
> *Hoangmai Pham (Chair)*, Institute for Exceptional Care
> *Margaret Chesney*, University of California, San Francisco
> *Deena Chisolm*, Nationwide Children's Hospital
> *David Erickson*, Federal Reserve Bank of New York
> *Christopher Koller*, Milbank Memorial Fund
> *Peter Long*, Blue Shield of California
> *L. Gordon Moore*, Goodside Health
> *Len M. Nichols*, The Urban Institute
> *Anaeze Offodile*, MD Anderson Cancer Center
> *Cheryl Powell*, Ad Hoc LLC
> *Joshua Sharfstein*, Johns Hopkins University
> *Dexter Shurney*, Adventist Health
> *Sarah Szanton*, Johns Hopkins University

reform but rather focuses on a cultural and movement-based shift away from economism and profits and toward valuing America's health in both numerical and cultural perspectives.

The report does not aim to present new governance, punitive, and accountability models or measures; dictate fiscal and monetary policy; discuss workforce or data issues; or suggest far-reaching changes such as a wholesale reform of public markets. Instead, the publication primarily aims to argue that, in absence of a legislative or government-based solution, health care, public health, and other stakeholders are obliged to act to the best of their ability. Therefore, the Steering Group intends this publication to be a call for a bottom-up movement to influence the nation writ large instead of a government-centric polemic.

DEFINITIONS

For the purposes of this Special Publication, the authors define **whole person health** as a person's ability to thrive and attain their full, optimized potential for health and well-being. Whole person health accounts for the whole person—not just separate organs or body systems—and considers the multiple factors that promote either health or disease. As depicted in Figure 1, whole person health necessitates helping and empowering individuals, families, communities,

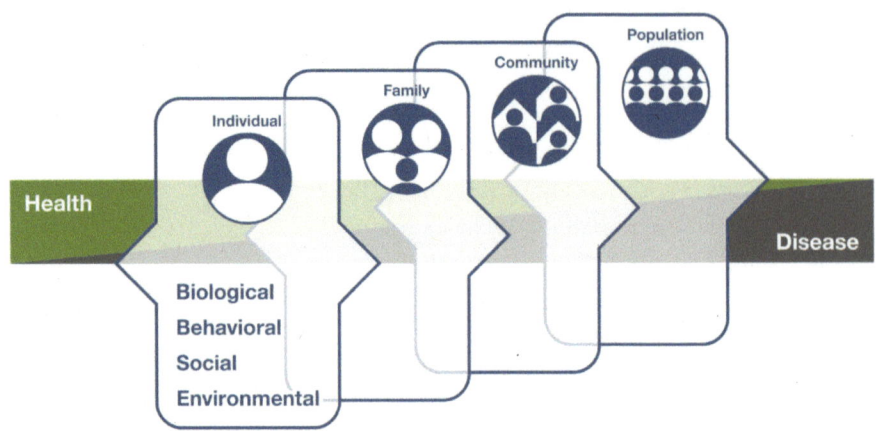

FIGURE 1 | Whole person health in the context of whole population health.
SOURCE: NCCIH, 2021.

and populations to improve their health in multiple interconnected biological, behavioral, social, and environmental arenas. Instead of limiting perspective to treatment of a specific disease, whole person health focuses on achieving, restoring, and maintaining health; promoting resilience; and preventing diseases across the life span. Whole person health defines the achievement of health and well-being by the conditions and criteria that individuals and communities identify as important.

The authors refer to **whole person, whole population health** as the extension of the focus of whole health to a group of people rather than just one individual. This may be viewed as conceptually distinct from traditional definitions of "population health," which are often primarily used for the purposes of attribution and geographic/demographic empanelment. For the purposes of this publication, **health and well-being** can be considered interchangeable with whole person, whole population health.

Whole person and whole population health care references clinical interventions that are based on the concept of whole person and whole population health and are:

1. grounded in personal health services oriented toward health promotion and prevention, in addition to treatment;
2. able to equitably enhance the health and well-being of an entire community or population;

3. person-centered rather than provider-centered;
4. relationship-based rather than transactional;
5. holistic, integrative, and continuous rather than fragmented and episodic; and
6. utilize measures that matter most to people, families, and populations, and support continuous learning and improvement in processes and structures that deliver better health, higher quality care, lower costs, and optimal individual and clinician experience.

For purposes of this Special Publication, the authors also wish to define and differentiate between health *financing* and health care *payment*. This Special Publication uses the term **health financing** to refer to the range of mechanisms through which improved health outcomes are targeted by funds that flow through various routes to support health, health care, social, environmental, and related services important to health. In health financing, money flows into the health and social services systems to fund and invest in activities and services known to improve health status, while **health care payment** is used to describe how service users and their fiduciary agents and insurers reimburse health providers for clinical and nonclinical interventions. For example, tax dollars and capital sources are health financing mechanisms, while mechanisms of health care payment include both fee-for-service structures (where clinicians and hospitals are paid for each service delivered) or prospective and value-based payment models.

CLARIFYING THE ROLE OF PRIVATE INVESTMENTS IN HEALTH AND HEALTH CARE

Throughout the Special Publication, the Steering Group calls for increasing private investments in health. While private equity has been labeled as a contributor to health inequities, the Steering Group believes that private investments can be a useful tool for the Special Publication's vision of whole person, whole population health if done in compliance with Securities and Exchange Commission investor protection and securities law. Private investments can also lead to more innovation in value-based health care models, yield important data on the time horizon and absolute returns of investments in whole health, and catalyze initiatives that seek to balance investment returns with broadly positive social and health impacts, such as the Collaborative Approach to Public Good Investments (CAPGI) or the Healthy Neighborhood Equity Funds (HNEFs).

REFERENCES

Morse, S. 2020. The Move to Value Accelerates in 2021, Spurred by Lack of Fee-for-Service Payments During Pandemic. Available at: https://www.healthcarefinancenews.com/news/move-value-accelerates-2021-spurred-lack-fee-service-payments-during-pandemic (accessed May 15, 2023).

NASEM (National Academies of Sciences, Engineering, and Medicine). 2021. *Financing That Rewards Better Health and Well-Being: Proceedings of a Workshop—in Brief.* Washington, DC: The National Academies Press. https://doi.org/10.17226/26332.

National Center for Complementary and Alternative Health. 2021. Whole Person Health: What You Need to Know. Available at: https://www.nccih.nih.gov/health/whole-person-health-what-you-need-to-know (accessed June 23, 2023).

1

VALUING AMERICA'S HEALTH

Our nation's health system[1] is failing. Between 2020 and 2022, more than 1 million Americans died from the COVID-19 pandemic (CDC, 2022). Due to the pandemic, in 2020, Americans experienced the largest 1-year drop in life expectancy since World War II (CDC, 2021a). Americans now have the lowest life expectancy observed since 2003, with structural racism driving even larger declines in life expectancy among Black and Latinx populations (Andrasfay and Goldman, 2021; CDC, 2022).

While uniquely devastating, the damage wrought by the pandemic belies a broader national health crisis. Before the pandemic, U.S. life expectancy fell from 2014 to 2015 and continued to decline through 2017—the longest sustained decline in life expectancy in a century (NASEM, 2021b). Additionally, our nation experiences the highest chronic disease burden among Organisation for Economic Co-operation and Development (OECD) countries, including the United Kingdom, France, and Germany (CDC, 2021c). The U.S. obesity rate, for example, is roughly two times that of our peer nations, on average.

Because of our high chronic disease prevalence, the United States experiences unusually high rates of avoidable and premature deaths, which has worsened over time and has disproportionately affected Black, Indigenous, and People of Color (BIPOC) populations due to structural racism (KFF, 2022; Tikkanen and Abrams, 2020). The number of reported pregnancy-related deaths in the United States has steadily increased from 7.2 deaths per 100,000 live births in 1987 to 17.3 deaths per 100,000 live births in 2017—the highest among OECD countries (CDC, 2021b; Tikkanen and Abrams, 2020). At the same time, Black women experienced a maternal mortality rate that is three and a half times more than that experienced by non-Hispanic White women and were five times more likely to die from pregnancy-related heart failure and blood pressure disorders (PRB, 2021).

---

[1] For the purposes of this publication, the term "health system" refers to the collective group of people, institutions, and resources that provide health care and related services in the United States.

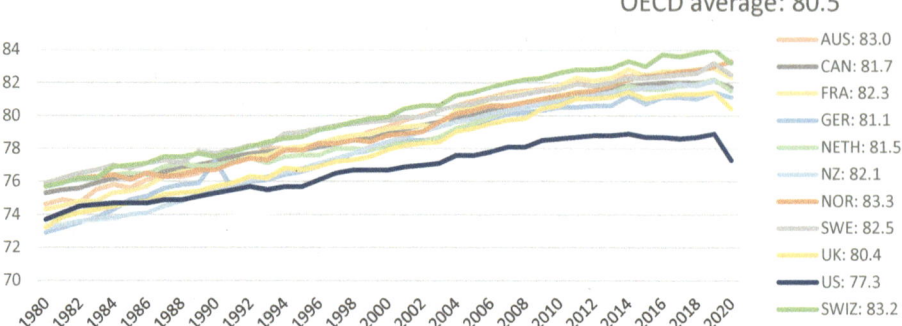

FIGURE 2 | Life expectancy for OECD countries.
NOTE: OECD average reflects the average of 38 OECD member countries, including ones not shown here.
SOURCE: OECD, 2022.

Our nation is also experiencing a crisis in mental health. Approximately 1 in 5 adults—nearly 50 million people—have experienced at least one mental illness, while more than 2.5 million youth report severe depression. Moreover, more than 60 percent of youth with severe depression do not receive treatment (Mental Health America, 2022). Thus, it is unsurprising that the United States reported the highest rates of death by suicide among OECD countries before the COVID-19 pandemic (Tiikanen and Abrams, 2020). Age-adjusted suicide rates increased 35 percent from 1999 to 2019, with an even higher increase (57 percent) in youth suicide rates from 2007 to 2018 (Curtin, 2020; SPRC, 2021). Furthermore, nearly 1 in 4 young girls have been found to self-harm, portending a protracted mental health crisis in the years to come (Pirani, 2018). Other deaths associated with feelings of despair have also occurred in shockingly high numbers. Driven by the opioid epidemic, where prescription painkillers were improperly approved, prescribed, and used, the number of drug overdose deaths has quadrupled since 1999, with nearly 500,000 individuals losing their lives to opioid overdoses (CDC, 2021c). The crisis continues to wreak havoc on the nation's social fabric, with illicit fentanyl and heroin continuing to cause avoidable deaths and secondary effects such as homelessness, unemployment, and school truancy (Feldscher, 2022). Overdoses are now a significant contributor to reductions in U.S. life expectancy, killing more Americans than suicides, motor vehicle accidents, firearms, and homicides (Graham, 2021). **The evidence of a national health crisis could not be clearer.**

Despite higher spending than any other OECD nation, at $4.1 trillion per year and growing, the U.S. health system is failing Americans through well-documented issues of unaffordability, inaccessibility, and disparities in care quality and access (CMS, 2021; Osborn et al., 2016; Schneider et al., 2021). Unfortunately, as much as one-third of these dollars are wasted due to the inefficiencies of the health care system. Care remains too expensive due to market failures and incentives that favor unnecessary, fragmented, or even harmful care, excessive prices, and administrative overhead. Meanwhile, programs and services that have been shown to maintain or improve health are woefully under-resourced (Berwick and Hackbarth, 2012).

The current trajectory of health spending, coupled with the nation's declining health status, is untenable and perilous. As evidenced by the COVID-19 pandemic, the systemic failure to invest adequately in a system that protects and promotes health led to disastrous outcomes in loss of life and economic productivity for individuals, families, and communities. These outcomes clearly demonstrate that—in both spending and practice— it is time to re-prioritize health and the services and interventions that advance it. Aligning financial incentives in ways that promote whole health across the life course requires a reimagination of how and what we pay for. Additionally, the nation will need to develop and implement innovative policies, clinical strategies, and new ways of investing in social, environmental, and community factors that change how we value[2] health.

A NEED FOR URGENT ACTION

The Steering Group recognizes that many efforts have centered on the need to transform health financing and health care payment from fee-for-service toward value-based care, including those led by nonprofit organizations, federal actors such as the Centers for Medicare & Medicaid Services (CMS) and the Center for Medicare & Medicaid Innovation (CMMI), and private players alike. While some improvement has been made over the past few decades, especially through the work led by CMMI, progress has largely been incremental. The lack of large-scale progress in transitioning from volume to value is not surprising, given that the status quo is quite profitable for many health care organizations and leaders (NAM, 2022). However, in light of the current negative trajectory of health in the United States and the profound impacts of a wasteful health system on

---

[2] The Steering Group largely defines value in health care through the prism of value-based care (i.e., exchange value). Health can also be improved by upstream social, environmental, and community factors that prevent disease and reduce morbidity incidence and prevalence, leading to reduced costs. Finally, the Special Publication defines value as an indicator of societal priorities (e.g., whether employers provide an environment and benefits that protect employee health, or whether the nation can accept the increasingly serious health impacts of racial and income inequality).

American society and well-being, the Steering Group believes that the time for incremental change is over.

By shining light on persistent inequities and vulnerabilities in the health and health care workforce and the crumbling public health infrastructure in the United States, COVID-19 has illustrated the dire consequences of not prioritizing health and the systems needed to maintain and promote it equitably across populations. Furthermore, our nation does not presently focus enough on the poorer outcomes of marginalized populations, especially along racial and ethnic lines but also including intersections across communities, identities, and factors including, but not limited to, sexual orientation and gender identity, income, and education. Finally, as experts in public health and health care, the Steering Group is concerned about the health and developmental outcomes in our nation's future—our children. We are alarmed by the high rates of childhood obesity and poverty, low social mobility and income stagnation, housing insecurity, and poor educational outcomes experienced by millions of American children. Because the Steering Group understands that health occurs on a continuum, with early childhood experiences substantially impacting health at every stage of life in increasingly compounding ways, we understand that transformation and change cannot wait.

The weight of these consequences necessitates the advocacy of patients, families, and communities to force urgent action by leaders in every sector—from the local to federal levels—to address existing and deepening health inequities and drive attention toward prioritizing health and tackling perverse incentives, market failures, and structural racism. Faced with the harrowing reality of the pandemic era, it is clear that investing time, finances, and collective efforts toward creating a healthier and more resilient system and populace is urgently needed. **But how do we, as stakeholders and leaders of the U.S. systems of health, health care, and biomedical science, approach and galvanize a broader movement to prioritize health? How do we invest in the strategies that build and protect it in a more equitable manner?**

The Steering Group looks to the example of climate change as both an inspiration and a model. Today, the global climate change movement is considered, perhaps, the world's most prominent social movement (Curran, 2015). Over the first two decades of the 21st century, a combination of public facilitators emphasized climate change as a critical global priority: the widespread impact of the 2006 film *The Inconvenient Truth* (Nolan, 2010); alarm from extreme hurricanes and wildfires across the United States; a global grassroots campaign led by youth activists and low-lying island nations (Daly, 2022; Witze, 2022); and renewable energy innovation (Eurasia Group, 2022).

Between 2019 and 2022, 3,135 companies across the globe committed to net-zero carbon by 2040—a bold, aggressive commitment that will require new investments, new technologies, change management, and broad-scale re-engineering and re-envisioning of how these organizations do business (The Climate Pledge, 2022). Those profiting from the status quo, such as fossil fuel companies, are not expected to lead a business transformation that has the potential to be financially damaging to them. Yet, these companies are slowly being pressured to join the many corporations working to shrink their carbon footprint. There is a growing recognition that addressing climate change is beneficial for all and that every economic and social sector should do its part. The need to address climate change has now experienced enough success and been viewed with enough urgency that, hopefully, decades of effort will make a meaningful impact.

While the climate change analogy has perhaps only partial applicability to the American health crisis, the issues identified by the Steering Group and the 2021 workshop described in Appendix A indicate that a similar approach and urgency is needed to address the nation's declining health status and worsening health inequities. The American health care system can no longer be looked to as the primary entity accountable to produce health for individuals and communities. It is often noted that, as currently structured, the American health care system pays for and profits from "sick care"—paying for illness and not for health—while the nation's public health system—which includes state and federal public health agencies and departments and is responsible for promoting health and well-being by preventing morbidity and mortality—has not been adequately funded or supported (Maani and Galea, 2020). Optimizing the effectiveness of this reactive method of improving individual and community health is, therefore, an inherently limited approach. Instead, similar to the climate change movement, the nation must elevate the goal of whole person population health across the life course as a priority far beyond the health care industry to include all sectors, including real estate that is affordable and equitably distributed and investments that reward the work of community-based organizations.

If leadership on prioritizing and producing health comes from empowered state, federal, and local actors, along with other non–health care system stakeholders (e.g., employers, investors, and entrepreneurs), the Steering Group believes that health care will eventually respond to new market demands and evolve to a system that profits from keeping people healthy as well as serving them when they are ill. In order to secure the cross-sector leadership and resources needed to invest in the mechanisms that we know can produce whole person health at scale, the circle of accountability for health must be broadened to reach far beyond the health care system. Collective accountability is not a revolutionary leap, as many entities are already invested in health in one form or another, ranging from U.S. taxpayers who are increasingly asked to fund ever more costly bills to sustain publicly supported health care, to employers who pay ever-increasing costs for sicker employees, and the many others who desire a more efficient and effective health system.

COVID-19 clearly demonstrated that, while everyone suffers from a sicker population, everyone can also benefit from a healthier society. This is because as societal conditions improve, the health and well-being benefits are experienced by everyone. The time has come for the United States to embrace these truths and take the long overdue steps to move away from incremental change and toward the bold action and leadership that is needed to propel our nation's health and health care system toward one that ensures better health for all. Just as businesses have committed to reducing their carbon footprint, the authors of this Special Publication hope to see organizations making commitments to improve the health of their employees and the communities in which they operate. Additionally, public and private resources should be redirected away from health care as we know it today, and toward those entities and programs that can improve and maintain health.

Just as COVID-19 demonstrated the need for urgent action, the national response to the crisis has shown us that rapid, meaningful change is possible where our priorities and purpose are clear and aligned. The speed of monumental actions undertaken to respond to COVID-19, including Operation Warp Speed, the rapid growth of telehealth, the unprecedented cross-sector collaboration among health care entities, strategically expanded scopes of practice, and the shifting of many services into the home, was previously considered impossible (NAM, 2022). As a nation, we must apply this same urgent and disruptive energy to the national crisis of declining American health to jolt us from our current course and reorient the nation on a path toward greater health and well-being. Our future and pre-eminence as a nation and world leader depend on it.

The insights included in this Special Publication provide both a vision for what a transformed U.S. health system could look like and key examples and strategies that stakeholders and leaders can use to progress. Chapter 2 describes six pillars of the transformative vision, while Chapter 3 details the elements of health care delivery and health financing models that have been successful in delivering, resourcing, and incentivizing whole person care, demonstrating that progress is already under way. Chapter 4 discusses priority actions that diverse stakeholders—including communities, government leaders, and private investors—can take to advance transformative efforts. These priority actions are intended to provide a useful, but not comprehensive, assessment of starting points for aligned action, acknowledging that other societal actors outside the scope of the Steering Group's expertise, such as education and law enforcement leaders, have a role to play as well. Lastly, Chapter 5 reiterates the need for disruptive change to achieve health transformation and provides examples of disruptive actions that can address upstream health determinants in a manner that is consistent with the vision and goals highlighted throughout the Special Publication.

REFERENCES

Andrasfay, T., and N. Goldman. 2021. Reductions in 2020 US life expectancy due to COVID-19 and the disproportionate impact on the Black and Latino populations. *Proceedings of the National Academy of Sciences* 118(5):e201476118. https://doi.org/10.1073/pnas.2014746118.

Bearden, T., H. L. Ratcliffe, J. R. Sugarman, A. Bitton, L. A. Anaman, G. Buckle, M. Cham, D. Chong Woei Quan, F. Ismail, B. Jargalsaikhan, W. Lim, N. M. Mohammad, I. C. N. Morrison, B. Norov, J. Oh, G. Riimaadai, S. Sararaks, and L. R. Hirschhorn. 2019. Empanelment: A foundational component of primary health care. *Gates Open Research* 3:1654. https://doi.org/10.12688/gatesopenres.13059.1.

Berwick, D. M., and A. D. Hackbarth. 2012. Eliminating waste in US health care. *JAMA* 307(14):1513-1516. https://doi.org/10.1001/jama.2012.362.

CDC (Centers for Disease Control and Prevention). 2021a. *Life Expectancy in the U.S. Declined a Year and Half in 2020.* Available at: https://www.cdc.gov/nchs/pressroom/nchs_press_releases/2021/202107.htm (accessed March 31, 2022).

CDC. 2021b. *Pregnancy Mortality Surveillance System.* Available at: https://www.cdc.gov/reproductivehealth/maternal-mortality/pregnancy-mortality-surveillance-system.htm (accessed March 31, 2022).

CDC. 2021c. *Understanding the Pandemic.* Available at: https://www.cdc.gov/drugoverdose/epidemic/index.html (accessed March 31, 2021).

CDC. 2022. *Risk for COVID-19 Infection, Hospitalization, and Death by Race/Ethnicity.* Available at: https://www.cdc.gov/coronavirus/2019-ncov/covid-data/investigations-discovery/hospitalization-death-by-race-ethnicity.html (accessed June 7, 2022).

Chua, P. S., J. Lee, and A. Anise, *rapporteurs.* 2022. *Multi-Payer Alignment on Value-Based Care.* Discussion Proceedings, National Academy of Medicine, Washington, DC. Available at: https://nam.edu/wp-content/uploads/2022/06/Multi-Payer-Alignment-on-Value-Based-Care-discussion-proceedings.pdf (accessed June 7, 2022).

CMS (Centers for Medicare & Medicaid Services). 2021. *National Health Expenditures 2020 Highlights.* Available at: https://www.cms.gov/files/document/highlights.pdf (accessed March 31, 2022).

Curran, G. 2015. Sustainability today: From fringe to mainstream. In *Sustainability and Energy Politics: Energy, Climate and the Environment.* Palgrave Macmillan, London. https://doi.org/10.1057/9781137352330_2.

Curtin, S. C. 2020. State suicide rates among adolescents and young adults aged 10-24: United States, 2000-2018. *National Vital Statistics Report* 69(11):1-9. Available at: https://www.cdc.gov/nchs/data/nvsr/nvsr69/nvsr-69-11-508.pdf (accessed March 31, 2022).

Daly, A. 2022. Climate competence: Youth climate activism and its impact on international human rights law. *Human Rights Law Review* 22:(2). https://doi.org/10.1093/hrlr/ngac011.

Eurasia Group. 2022. *Top Risks 2022.* Available at: https://www.eurasiagroup.net/files/upload/EurasiaGroup_TopRisks2022.pdf (accessed June 7, 2022).

Feldscher, K. 2022. *What Led to the Opioid Crisis—and How to Fix it.* Available at: https://www.hsph.harvard.edu/news/features/what-led-to-the-opioid-crisis-and-how-to-fix-it (accessed January 23, 2022).

Graham, C. 2021. *America's Crisis of Despair: A Federal Task Force for Economic Recovery and Societal Well-Being.* Available at: https://www.brookings.edu/research/americas-crisis-of-despair-a-federal-task-force-for-economic-recovery-and-societal-well-being (accessed June 6, 2022).

KFF. 2022. *Key Facts on Health and Health Care by Race and Ethnicity.* Available at: https://www.kff.org/report-section/key-facts-on-health-and-health-care-by-race-and-ethnicity-health-status-outcomes-and-behaviors (accessed January 3, 2023).

Maani, S., and S. Galea 2020. COVID-19 and underinvestment in the public health infrastructure of the United States. *The Millbank Quarterly* 98(2):250-259. https://doi.org/10.1111/1468-0009.12463.

Mental Health America. 2022. *The State of Mental Health in America.* Available at: https://www.mhanational.org/issues/state-mental-health-america (accessed July 19, 2022).

Morse, S. 2020. The Move to Value Accelerates in 2021, Spurred by Lack of Fee-for-Service Payments During Pandemic. Available at: https://www.healthcarefinancenews.com/news/move-value-accelerates-2021-spurred-lack-fee-service-payments-during-pandemic (accessed May 15, 2023).

NAM (National Academy of Medicine). 2022. *Emerging Stronger from COVID-19: Priorities for Health System Transformation.* A. Anise, L. Adams, M. Ahmed, A. Bailey, P. S. Chua, C. S. Chukwurah, M. Cocchiola, A. Cupito, K. Kadakia, J.

Lee, and A. Williams, *editors*. NAM Special Publication. Washington, DC: The National Academies Press. https://doi.org/10.17226/26657.

NASEM (National Academies of Sciences, Engineering, and Medicine). 2021a. *Financing That Rewards Better Health and Well-Being: Proceedings of a Workshop—in Brief.* Washington, DC: The National Academies Press. https://doi.org/10.17226/26332.

NASEM. 2021b. *High and Rising Mortality Rates Among Working-Age Adults.* Washington, DC: The National Academies Press. https://doi.org/10.17226/25976.

Nolan, J. M. 2010. "An inconvenient truth" increases knowledge, concern, and willingness to reduce greenhouse gases. *Environment and Behavior* 42(5):643-658. https://doi.org/10.1177/0013916509357696.

Osborn, R., D. Squires, M. M. Doty, D. O. Sarnak, and E. C. Schneider. 2016. In new survey of eleven countries, US adults still struggle with access to and affordability of health care. *Health Affairs* 35(12):2327-2336. https://doi.org/10.1377/hlthaff.2016.1088.

Pirani, F. 2018. *Nearly 1 in 4 Teen Girls in the US Self-Harm, Massive High School Survey Finds.* Available at: https://www.ajc.com/news/health-med-fit-science/nearly-teen-girls-the-self-harm-massive-high-school-survey-finds/EQnLJy3REFX53HjbHGnukJ (accessed January 24, 2023).

PRB (Population Reference Bureau). 2021. *Black Women Over Three Times More Likely to Die in Pregnancy, Postpartum Than White Women, New Research Finds.* Available at: https://www.prb.org/resources/black-women-over-three-times-more-likely-to-die-in-pregnancy-postpartum-than-white-women-new-research-finds (accessed January 23, 2022).

Schneider, E., A. Shah, M. M. Doty, R. Tikkanen, K. Fields, and R. D. Williams. 2021. *Mirror, Mirror 2021: Reflecting Poorly.* The Commonwealth Fund. Available at: https://www.commonwealthfund.org/publications/fund-reports/2021/aug/mirror-mirror-2021-reflecting-poorly (accessed March 31, 2022).

SPRC (Suicide Prevention Resource Center). 2021. *Suicide Mortality in the U.S., 1999–2019.* https://sprc.org/news/suicide-mortality-us-1999-2019 (accessed March 31, 2022).

The Climate Pledge. 2022. *Net-Zero Carbon by 2040.* Available at: https://www.theclimatepledge.com (accessed June 8, 2022).

Tikkanen, R., and M. K. Abrams. 2020. *U.S. Health Care from a Global Perspective, 2019: Higher Spending, Worse Outcomes?* The Commonwealth Fund. Available at: https://www.commonwealthfund.org/publications/issue-briefs/2020/jan/us-health-care-global-perspective-2019 (accessed March 31, 2022).

Verweij M., and A. Daweson. 2020. Sharing responsibility: Responsibility for health is not a zero-sum game. *Public Health Ethics* 12(2):99-102. https://doi.org/10.1093/phe/phz012.

Witze, A. 2022. Climate change—four decades of missed opportunities. *Nature* 604(7905):239-240. https://doi.org/10.1038/d41586-022-00998-4.

2

A VISION FOR BETTER HEALTH AND WELL-BEING

Bridging the gap between the inefficient, ineffective, and inequitable realities of the current U.S. health system and the strategies needed to achieve better health and well-being requires a bold, disruptive, yet realistic vision for a transformed health system. This vision must be grounded in the principles of person-centricity, cross-sector collaboration (as described in Chapters 3 and 4), and equity.

With these principles at the center, the vision can inspire financial strategies that will sustainably resource, incentivize, and deliver health system transformation. For this vision to come to fruition, every stakeholder invested in ensuring better health has the responsibility to enact short-term repairs, mid-term renovations, and long-term redesigns in multiple sectors across the health system for decades to come. The key pillars of this vision, as conceived by the Steering Group, are presented in Box 2 and described in the text that follows.

1. U.S. health status is at least that of other middle- and high-income countries, with inequities eliminated.

While the United States spends the most on health care compared to other Organisation for Economic Co-operation and Development (OECD) countries and ranks high for scientific and clinical innovation as well as survival rates for some cancers, it has the lowest life expectancy, highest chronic disease incidence, and the poorest health outcomes (Peter G. Peterson Foundation, 2022; Tikkanen and Abrams, 2020). This contradiction indicates that our nation does not provide an equivalent level of equitable, efficient, or effective conditions to promote whole person, whole population health as its peer nations. The first step toward realizing the Steering Group's vision is to ensure U.S. health status is at least that of or exceeds other OECD countries through the pillars, goals, and actions suggested throughout this Special Publication.

> **BOX 2**
>
> *Key Pillars of the Vision for Whole Person and Whole Population Health and Well-Being*
>
> 1. U.S. health status is at least that of other middle- and high-income countries, with inequities eliminated.
> 2. Health and health equity are nationwide commitments spanning beyond organizations in health care and public health.
> 3. Health care expenditures as a percentage of the gross domestic product (GDP) do not constrain and displace other important social services that directly impact health and equity.
> 4. Economic and cultural incentives encourage every stakeholder sector to take health promoting actions and make health promoting investments.
> 5. Efforts from all sectors, including government programs and regulations, are organized to prioritize the health of individuals, communities, and society.
> 6. Individuals and communities are empowered as organization and delivery decision-makers for matters pertaining to their health.

This process will primarily include rallying a whole-of-society approach, including but not limited to health care and public health systems, to target the drivers of the rapid, inequitable, and sustained decrease in U.S. life expectancy. In many instances, poor health in America has been driven by growing and intersecting inequities in care and outcomes, driven by racial, ethnic, socioeconomic, disability, and geographic factors, over time (IOM, 2003).

The high prevalence of morbidity and mortality discussed in Chapter 1 reflects the impact of inequities in the drivers of health as well as the structural racism that established and continues to enable these injustices. Structural racism is a fundamental driver of health disparities in the United States, with a system that reinforces and restricts opportunities for long, healthy lives of Black Americans and other people of color. This discrimination and injustice manifests and intersects with the drivers of health: quality housing and neighborhoods, access to economic opportunities, quality education, and health care (Churchwell et al., 2020). Thus, America must not only reckon with—and reform systems and structures to improve—overall population health, but also structural racism in order to improve the nation's health. This transformation will require considerable effort in domains upstream or adjacent to health care and public health systems, including housing, food, transportation, education, employment, and public safety (Churchwell et al., 2020).

Tackling structural racism must also work hand in hand with the key structural economic issue of wealth inequality and poverty. In the United States, only 2 percent of household wealth is held by the bottom 50 percent of households. This disparity is exacerbated by systemic and structural racism, resulting in the average American Black family having eight times less wealth than the average American White family. On a broader population level, 36 percent of all Americans have no savings at all, and another 19 percent have less than $1,000 saved (Bieber, 2023). The consequences of this lack of wealth are manifested on a developmental level, with less wealthy individuals at greater risk for exposure to damaging air pollution (as a result of residential segregation or low quality of housing), lower educational attainment and achievement, violence and homicide, risk of developing and dying from a chronic disease, and, ultimately, lower life expectancy (Avanceña et al., 2021). This higher mortality occurs due to a constellation of risk factors that comes from the psychosocial anxiety and stress of inequality: People with low incomes are more likely to smoke, consume an unhealthy diet due to poverty and food insecurity, experience unemployment and job security, and are two times as likely to die from sudden health incidents (Avanceña et al., 2021).

To realize the Steering Group's vision of whole person, whole population health, there must be a bottom-up, community-led movement that involves aligning the forces of institutions that reinforce racial discrimination, perpetuate wealth inequality and poverty, and drive adverse health outcomes from the prenatal or developmental stage throughout the entire life course (Bailey et al., 2017). These institutions include, but are not limited to, education, banking, media, criminal justice, and health care.

A transformed health system that achieves whole person and whole population health and well-being can only exist when every person has the opportunity, resources, and support to achieve their best health, with particular attention and actions targeted to those most in need. To advance health equity, we must expand our collective notion of the sources and drivers of health, as well as design systems and make efforts to address health and health-related social needs at their inception. It is only by taking intentional and systemic action that we can radically, and uniformly, improve America's health.

2. Health and health equity are nationwide commitments spanning beyond organizations in health care and public health.

For many years, it has been broadly accepted that health care is responsible for contributing only a minority of what it takes to produce overall health, while social and economic factors, income, genetic predisposition, and personal lifestyle choices are much more influential (Braveman and Gottlieb, 2014). Despite this understanding, the health care sector is still prioritized as the source of accountability and leadership for health outcomes, regardless of the suitability of state, local, tribal, and territorial health departments to serve as backbone organizations for cross-sector partnerships to address the social determinants of health. Therefore, the resources and infrastructure necessary for public health departments to succeed are often absent, severely limiting the ability of public health entities to coordinate public health responses and facilitate broad multi-stakeholder collaboration that could help decentralize governance of and accountability for health (Galea and Maani, 2020).

The disconnect between underinvesting in public health and over-allocating resources to the health care sector reflects a lack of policy coherence in the nation; financing is not distributed so that health care, public health, and other health promoting sectors such as housing, social services, and food interact and synergize to promote population health and health equity. The first priority of realizing the goal of whole person, whole population health should be to implement the principle of "health in every policy" and apply this principle consistently. An example of this change would be a national health infrastructure that integrates stronger public health systems. Adequately funding public health would build the capability to collect, analyze, and apply data, reduce inequities in health care and public health system capacity, and strengthen the role of individuals, families, and communities as leaders in promoting whole person, whole population health. The system would then be able to effectively prevent disease and promote health, detect emerging health crises, and maintain the ability to respond to noncommunicable and infectious disease threats.

Another disconnect is the de-emphasized priority of health in economic decision-making. Business and economic decisions are often incentivized by financial priorities measured through growth and profit-driven metrics such as, but not limited to, revenue growth, total shareholder returns, or return on equity (Bradley et al., 2022). The consequence of these incentives is a mindset highlighted in several examples below, that has negatively impacted the nation's health by ignoring potential harm in favor of financial gain:

- A company deciding to market and sell unhealthy food and beverages to children (e.g., large portion sizes, products with high levels of sugar and sodium) adversely affecting their diets across the life course;
- Land developers and zoning boards deciding to exclude walkable and outdoor spaces in urban areas because they could reduce profits;

- A local government administrator deprioritizing lowering barriers to constructing affordable housing;
- A policy maker voting to restrict access to preventive care for low-income families; or
- Hospital system leadership deciding to construct an additional facility rather than invest in upstream interventions that would disrupt existing structural barriers and improve the baseline health of patients.

Furthermore, existing policy interventions that promote health in economic decisions are often unevenly applied. While building a new road or structure typically requires a corporation to submit an environmental impact assessment, similar discussions or assessments on health impact are infrequent and nonstandard. Changing this disconnect to promote the careful consideration of health impact in a similar manner to how potential environmental impact is currently considered would ensure more responsibility for the tremendous power that business decisions have on communities, families, and futures across our nation.

This change must begin through cross-sector cooperation and collaboration, which could be accomplished if policy makers adopt whole person, whole population health as the primary framework on which the United States will develop into the future. This framework could be applied through funding and accountability actions such as, but not limited to, legislating new policies and programs at the federal and state levels; creating and enforcing health, environmental, and financial sector regulations within government agencies; and devising incentives that encourage capital allocation that contribute a net social positive to whole person, whole population health throughout the nation.

Several recent programs, policies, and legislation would fit such a framework. These include the 2022 Inflation Reduction Act, which enabled the government to negotiate for lower prescription prices for Medicaid and incentivized renewable energy and electric vehicles (Cabral and Sherman, 2022). Other examples include the Safer Communities Act, which appropriated $250 million for states to expand community mental health services and an additional $240 million over 4 years for mental health awareness among school-aged youth, including training for school personnel and other adults. At the state level, policies that could improve health outcomes include increasing the minimum wage, which has been linked with a decrease in infant mortality and low weight births and has significant health dividends across the life course (Avanceña et al., 2021). Other solutions that tackle structural drivers of poor health across the life course include reducing barriers to access for the Supplemental Nutrition Assistance Program and expanding Medicaid benefits under the Affordable Care Act (Carlson and Llobrera, 2022;

Leigh and Du, 2018; NIMHD, 2022). Finally, expanding programs such as the Earned Income Tax credit but also focusing on other strategies that promote employment and increase parental income could help dismember some aspects of structural racism by promoting intervention at the household level (Gitterman et al., 2016).

Additionally, current Securities and Exchange Commission efforts to enhance the transparency of Environmental, Social, and Governance (ESG) screening methodologies for finance and investment products will promote additional capital flows into companies that contribute to the social good, although they took 30 years to put into place (U.S. Securities and Exchange Commission, 2022). Finally, the expanded Child Tax Credit, despite ending after its 1-year authorization from the 2021 American Rescue Plan Act ended, lifted 3.7 million children out of poverty and provided improved nutrition, decreased reliance on credit cards, and enhanced access to education (Hamilton et al., 2022). These policies highlight that, if consistent and sustained legislation, investments, and regulations with health as the priority are applied, it would radically transform the nation's health toward the Steering Group's vision of whole person, whole population health.

3. Health care expenditures as a percentage of the GDP do not constrain and displace other important social services that directly impact health and equity.

The current proportion of the GDP spent on health expenditures is unsustainable. In 2020, health care expenditures accounted for 19.7 percent of the U.S. GDP (CMS, 2020). This figure has more than tripled since 1960, with health care expenditure increases outpacing the growth rates of GDP, inflation, and population across the same period (Nunn and Shambaugh, 2020).

While the status of the United States as a wealthy nation with an aging population accounts for some of this growth, the pace and nature indicate a highly unsustainable fiscal situation relative to undesirable health care costs and health outcomes (Peter G. Peterson Foundation, 2022). At the federal and state levels, rising health expenditures combined with worsening health outcomes reflect wasteful government spending that, with needed adjustments and alterations, could be lessened with vastly improved outcomes.

U.S. health care expenditures grew from $2.6 trillion in 2010 to $3.65 trillion in 2018 (Antos and Capretta, 2020). Over roughly the same period (2008-2018), public health spending experienced no statistically significant growth (with the exception of spending on injury prevention), hovering around $93 billion annually (Alfonso et al., 2021). This substantial gap indicates misplaced priorities that emphasize a reactive sick-care approach to health instead of a system that espouses the preventive and health-promoting aspects of whole person, whole population health. By underinvesting in policies and programs that improve the overall health and well-being of populations and instead allocating funding to sick care, the interventions that could target drivers of structural inequality, poverty, and racism are neglected. Shifting investments toward public health interventions, programs, and policies as well as targeting high-impact areas, such as the social drivers of health and structural racism, could rapidly improve overall health and well-being (Kindig, 2022). Efforts could include employment opportunities focused on reducing structural inequality, including reducing discrimination in the workplace, increasing accessibility to nutritious and less calorie-dense diets, and instituting policies to expand housing access that also dismantle segregation across economic and racial lines, among many others (Churchwell et al., 2020). These investments would ultimately reduce the need and, therefore, the cost of sick care.

Rising health care costs will continue to impact American employers and households unless health system transformation as outlined in this Special Publication occurs. Despite growing insurance coverage and out-of-pocket cost reductions provided by the Affordable Care Act, the share of household spending attributed to health care in the United States increased from 5.9 percent in 2004 to 8.1 percent in 2018 (Chalise, 2020). Out-of-pocket payments for medical services, drugs, and supplies accounted for roughly one-third of household health care expenditures in 2018 and health insurance (which largely reflects the underlying cost of medical care due to medical loss ratios capping administrative costs and profit) consumed the remaining two-thirds, indicating that medical (i.e., sick-care) costs directly and indirectly drive households' increasing health care spending (Chalise, 2018). Since 2011, health insurance premiums and deductibles have climbed substantially, with average monthly premiums increasing from $217 in 2011 to $515 in 2019 (reflecting 11.6 percent growth per year). The average deductible for an average plan offered on Healthcare.gov has also increased, from $2,425 in 2011 to $4,500 in 2020 (Antos and Capretta, 2020). If health care cost increases had aligned with the growth in the Consumer Price Index, an average American family would save approximately $553 per month, yielding roughly $6,636 annually to spend on other needs and priorities (BLS, 2022).

The solution to rising health care costs is complex and difficult to solve. There are substantial incentives and underlying market power of health care system actors to set elevated health care prices (NASI, 2015). At nearly one-fifth of the U.S. economy, health care actors and their investors often pursue commercial interests, such as increasing rates, resisting participation in value-based care models, and streamlining operations to produce favorable quarterly earnings and distributions for shareholders. These rational actions result in the collective dysfunction of the U.S. health and health care system, including sub-optimal care outcomes and high costs (Chua et al., 2022). Furthermore, the political and economic influence of the health care industry combined with the complexity of the U.S. health care system increases the difficulty of devising coherent solutions to transition to value-based care and improve care quality and outcomes (King, 2017; Wang and Anderson, 2022).

While lowering high health care prices by targeting market power and perverse incentives is a worthy goal that may reduce waste and enhance health care quality, this solution would not fully solve the declining health status of all Americans. Instead, the best and most effective way for the United States to spend less on health care and ensure whole person, whole population health is to create the conditions by which people and populations can be healthy, with as little intervention from health care as possible.

4. Economic and cultural incentives encourage every stakeholder sector to take health promoting actions and make health promoting investments.

Fully optimizing health and well-being in the United States also necessitates economic incentives and societal norms that reinforce the vision. To accelerate the transformative progress needed, the Steering Group envisions a future in which policies incentivize health promotion and disincentivize harmful activities and exist alongside widespread social consensus on the importance of whole person and whole population health and well-being.

Drawing again on ongoing work in reducing the impact of climate change, some governments have exceeded commitments made in the Paris Climate Agreement by joining a whole-of-society approach to addressing climate change with laws and policies that disincentivize carbon emissions (Mora, 2013). This combination of public accountability, regulatory factors, and societal pressure has led some entities to take even larger strides toward the end goal, with corporations like Google and Microsoft aiming to be "carbon negative" and powered by renewable energy by 2030.

Achieving a transformed state of health and well-being in the United States will require a combination of societal and economic interventions as part of a broader movement to prioritize a holistic conception of health. The public must be able to expect that employers would prioritize the physical and mental health, social cohesion, and well-being of their employees by creating healthy workplaces and cultures, including the provision of a living wage. Public health departments must be adequately funded to perform their core functions of resource coordination, stakeholder alignment, surveillance and monitoring, needs assessment, disease prevention, and health promotion to meet 21st-century needs. Institutions such as schools must be on the front lines of tackling structural racism, poverty, and inequality and promoting whole person, whole population health at an early stage of life. Schools and other educational institutions could promote health literacy, ensuring access to healthy food, encouraging physical fitness, and protecting students from violence and harmful influences. At all ages, especially from early childhood, providing opportunities for social-emotional learning—a pedagogical method for developing self-awareness, self-control, and interpersonal skills—could form the basis of life-long resilience and success in health. This approach could also improve academic performance, reduce bullying, and lower drop-out rates (Committee for Children, 2022).

Given the benefits of a whole-of-society approach for communities and corporations, individual and collective investments must be made to empower and advance a social infrastructure that will enable the creation of a public health and health care system that promotes and enables whole person, whole population health. Policies should also support and reward health promoting investments through grants, tax breaks, and incentives that share costs between governments, communities, and responsible organizations to promote health. Moving forward, both social and economic considerations and pressures must be aligned to create demand for new and better solutions. Federal and state policy makers should appropriate more impactful health-enhancing investments and enact financial and reputational penalties for actions and practices that harm the public's health.

5. Efforts from all sectors, including government programs and regulations, are organized to prioritize the health of individuals, communities, and society.

Government programs and funding streams are not currently structured to promote whole health for individuals or populations. The distribution of services among multiple agencies, inconsistencies in policy, and uneven funding leads to silos and inefficiencies in the financing and organization of services and can even serve to worsen individual and community health.

The Steering Group envisions a transformed health system where public and community-based programs and services are designed to maximize individual, family, and community health and well-being. This transformation must also help ensure that those who have been historically marginalized can efficiently and effectively access well-resourced and equitably designed interventions that support whole person, whole population health and well-being, including economic and social support interventions. Aligned with a diverse array of community needs and informed by individual engagement (discussed in the section below), the services most essential for producing health and well-being must be appropriately funded and sustainably incentivized to ensure reliable and equitable service provision for individuals, families, and communities. These interventions would reduce the negative life-long impacts of poverty, material deprivation, and inequality. Based on their long-term and reliable relationship to better health, examples of these services may include investments in state, local, tribal, and territorial public health workforce development, programs, and services; access to affordable housing; expansion of home- and community-based services; investments in preschool and early childhood care and education, as well as K-12 education; strengthened employment assistance; and Supplemental Nutrition Assistance Program (SNAP) assistance.

Under the Steering Group's vision, programs such as these would be applied on a broader scale to ensure that beneficiaries can access what they need to improve their health efficiently, affordably, and equitably and choose the interventions that would help them the most. These interventions include the ability to access public health insurance or SNAP through a "no-wrong-door" approach or recent efforts in Arkansas, Massachusetts, and Oregon leveraging Medicaid 1115 waivers to develop food-as-medicine initiatives that expanded access to food tailored to individual medical needs, nutrition counseling, and even cooking classes (Held, 2022). The full realization of this aspect of the vision would result in the incorporation of health in every policy, with government at all levels focused on the equitable provision of health across their respective jurisdictions. Grants, funding, and policies across all agencies would be evaluated for their potential to advance a broad conception of health and, wherever possible, redesigned to ensure better health equity and the health of individuals and communities.

6. Individuals and communities are empowered as organization and delivery decision-makers for matters pertaining to their health.

Determining the best way to measure the construct of health as "a state of physical, social, and emotional well-being, not just the absence of disease" remains challenging (WHO, 2022). Two critical elements of importance to individuals and communities are engagement in determining measures of success in health care and recognition as decision-makers related to investments intended to benefit their health.

Current health care measurement models—largely rooted in Donabedian's model, which analyzes quality via structure, process, and outcomes—overemphasize clinical and process-based outcome measures (Donabedian, 1988). The implication of this framework is the widespread adoption of the accountability approach to creating measures, which emphasizes the measurement, incentivization, and rewarding of a series of functional and clinical processes and outcomes. Our current health care payment system, including the Centers for Medicare & Medicaid Services, has largely endorsed the use of these models to assess health system performance as well as outcomes and, therefore, drive payment (NAM, 2022).

This approach largely neglects core elements of whole person, whole population health, such as patient and family engagement in care delivery and consideration of the long-term health and well-being of individuals and populations served, as opposed to relatively short-term clinical outcomes. For example, at a systems level, the breadth and depth of measurement requirements have led to a suboptimal allocation of resources, prioritizing administrative data and electronic medical record collection activities and requirements over providing services that benefit whole-person, whole-population health and well-being. This system has also led to significant clinician burnout that further harms individuals by limiting opportunities to access care (Shah et al., 2020).

Developing a system that supports whole person, whole population health will require a novel and disruptive redesign in health care payment and financing, fueled by creative, person-centric approaches to measuring success, such as prioritization of patient-identified goals at the point-of-care (e.g., being able to walk their daughter down the aisle in 3 months' time) and disparity reduction, over some of the more traditional performance measures.

Engagement of individuals and communities should not only be restricted to measurement and payment. The vision of whole person, whole population health also advocates for a disruptive transformation in resource allocation and investments in health that is led by communities and individuals. Under the vision, the Steering Group determined that communities and individuals within localities know best regarding the services that would have the most significant impact on their health. As such, they should be central participants in decision-making processes that purport to invest in their health (Singletary and Chin, 2023).

Both key elements for meaningful engagement—community-driven measures to define success and drive payment, as well as community-driven allocation of resources and investment in health—would represent a radical shift from the status quo. Under a transformed whole health system, communities and individuals would participate in defining, measuring, and investing in the necessary components, services, and programs that would enable them to realize their fullest potential health.

CONCLUSION

What can be learned from other effective social change movements in American history, such as the civil rights movement and climate change? What elements are needed to kick-start and maintain a movement to prioritize the health and well-being of the population? In 2013, the National Academies' Roundtable on Population Health Improvement sponsored a workshop to explore the lessons gleaned from social movements to accelerate a movement to improve health and promote health equity (IOM, 2014). A key message from that workshop is that "social movements emerge from the efforts of purposeful actors, individuals, or organizations to respond to changes [and] conditions experienced as unjust—to assert new public values, form new relationships, and mobilize political, economic, and cultural power to translate those values into action" (IOM, 2014, p. 10). Social movements must also incorporate goals, leadership, strategy, structure, and effective messaging while allowing for organic relationships and communities of practice that breed transformative influence far greater than the sum of individual contributions (Wheatley and Frieze, 2006). Successful movements also often take advantage of political opportunities to enact change. Additionally, effective health-related movements in the past often had an antagonist—such as "Big Tobacco" during the anti-smoking movement—that helped coalesce and sharpen efforts (Yale University, 2022).

After examining the characteristics of successful social movements of the past, it appears that critical elements may already be in place for the movement to prioritize whole person, whole population health, well-being, and equity to synergize with the nation's reckoning with structural racism and wealth inequality. The nation and the world are emerging from a devastating era marked by disease and death, as the COVID-19 pandemic has taken more than a million lives with a disproportionate impact on communities of color, people with disabilities, and the socioeconomically disadvantaged (Andrasfay and Goldman, 2021; CDC, 2022). The murder of George Floyd on May 25, 2020, escalated calls for racial and social justice and called attention to the deep disparities that have persisted in the U.S. health system for decades. The pandemic also demonstrated that rapid change is possible by stimulating new norms for vaccine development, information sharing, telecommuting, and virtual health care to meet a moment of crisis.

To ensure the United States reaches the north star—a whole person, whole population health system—the nation must sustain the disruption of current systems with the forcefulness and urgency of the contemporary social movements of the past several decades. The imperative should not be to avert or respond to our health crisis. Instead, we must first repair systemic and structural failures to ensure U.S. health status matches or exceeds that of other OECD nations. Second, every stakeholder, company, and entity must be held accountable and responsible for overall health and health equity in the nation. Third, health care expenditures must be contained, with a more equitable allocation to public health systems given their core mission of health promotion and disease prevention. Fourth, clear economic and cultural incentives are needed to encourage every sector that benefits from improved health to embrace health promoting actions and investments. Fifth, a collaborative financing and policy-making approach, from government regulations, new legislation, and the reconceptualization of economic success, is required to enable change that prioritizes whole person, whole population health. Finally, individuals and communities must be able to use their knowledge, power, and autonomy to direct decisions about health services, processes, and infrastructure that are most meaningful to them.

The next chapter further illustrates the need for disruptive, transformational action through case studies on innovative care models and interventions. Despite the rapid innovation, pilots, and successes of these models, the chapter also illustrates their limited impact relative to the scale and severity of the current national health crisis.

REFERENCES

Alfonso, Y. N., J. P. Leider, B. Resnick, J. M. McCullough, and D. Bishai. 2021. US public health neglected: Flat or declining spending left states ill equipped to respond to COVID-19. *Health Affairs* 40(4):664-671. https://doi.org/10.1377/hlthaff.2020.01084.

Antos, J. R., and J. C. Capretta. 2020. The ACA: Trillions? Yes. A Revolution? No. *Health Affairs* April. https://doi.org/10.1377/forefront.20200406.93812.

Avanceña, A. L. V., E. K. DeLuca, B. Lott, A. Mauri, N. Miller, D. Eisenberg, and D. W. Hutton. 2021. Income and income inequality are a matter of life and death: What can policymakers do about it? *American Journal of Public Health* 111:1404-1408. https://doi.org/10.2105/AJPH.2021.306301.

Bailey, Z. D., N. Krieger, M. Agénor, J. Graves, N. Linos, and M. T. Bassett. 2017. Structural racism and health inequities in the USA: Evidence and interventions. *The Lancet* 389(10077):1453-1463. https://doi.org//10.1016/s0140-6736(17)30569-x.

Bieber, C. 2023. *Americans Do Not Have Enough Savings. Here's What You Can Do About It.* Available at: https://www.nasdaq.com/articles/americans-do-not-have-enough-savings.-heres-what-you-can-do-about-it (accessed May 15, 2023).

BLS (U.S. Bureau of Labor Statistics). 2022. *Consumer Price Index for All Urban Consumers: Medical Care in U.S. City Average.* Available at: https://fred.stlouisfed.org/series/CPIMEDSL (accessed October 6, 2022).

Bradley, C., R. Doherty, N. Northcote, and T. Röder. 2022. *The Ten Rules of Growth.* McKinsey. Available at: https://www.mckinsey.com/capabilities/strategy-and-corporate-finance/our-insights/the-ten-rules-of-growth (accessed October 5, 2022).

Braveman, P., and L. Gottlieb. 2014. The social determinants of health: It's time to consider the causes of the causes. *Public Health Reports* 129(1 Suppl 2):19-31.

Cabral, S., and N. Sherman. 2022. *Biden Signs Climate, Tax and Health Bill into Law.* Available at: https://www.bbc.com/news/world-us-canada-62568772 (accessed October 11, 2022).

Carlson, S., and J. Llobrera. 2022. *SNAP Is Linked with Improved Health Outcomes and Lower Health Care Costs.* Available at: https://www.cbpp.org/research/food-assistance/snap-is-linked-with-improved-health-outcomes-and-lower-health-care-costs (accessed February 16, 2023).

Chalise, L. 2020. *How Have Healthcare Expenditures Changed? Evidence from the Consumer Expenditure Surveys.* Available at: https://www.bls.gov/opub/btn/volume-9/how-have-healthcare-expenditures-changed-evidence-from-the-consumer-expenditure-surveys.htm (accessed October 7, 2020).

Chua, P. S., J. Lee, and A. Anise, *rapporteurs.* 2022. *Multi-Payer Alignment on Value-Based Care.* Discussion Proceedings. Washington, DC: National Academy of Medicine. Available at: https://nam.edu/wp-content/uploads/2022/06/Multi-Payer-Alignment-on-Value-Based-Care-discussion-proceedings.pdf (accessed June 7, 2022).

Churchwell, K., M. S. V. Elkind, R. M. Benjamin, A. P. Carson, E. K. Chang, W. Lawrence, A. Mills, T. M. Odom, C. J. Rodriguez, F. Rodriguez, E. Sanchez, A. Z. Sharrief, M. Sims, O. Williams, and American Heart Association. 2020. Call to action: Structural racism as a fundamental driver of health disparities: A presidential advisory from the American Heart Association. *Circulation* 142(24):e454-e468. https://doi.org/10.1161/0000000000000936.

CMS (Centers for Medicare & Medicaid Services). 2021. *National Health Expenditures 2020 Highlights.* Available at: https://www.cms.gov/files/document/highlights.pdf (accessed March 31, 2022).

Committee for Children. 2022. *What Is Social-Emotional Learning? Helping Everyone Thrive.* Available at: https://www.cfchildren.org/what-is-social-emotional-learning (accessed June 9, 2022).

Donabedian, A. 1988. The quality of care: How can it be assessed? *JAMA* 260(12):1743-1748. https://doi.org/10.1001/jama.260.12.1743.

Gitterman, B. A., P. J. Flanagan, W. H. Cotton, K. J. Dilley, J. H. Duffee, A. E. Green, V. A. Keane, S. D. Krugman, J. M. Linton, C. D. McKelvey, and J. L. Nelson. 2016. Poverty and child health in the United States. *Pediatrics* 137(4):e20160339. https://doi.org/10.1542/peds.2016-0339.

Hamilton, L., S. Roll, M. Despard, E. Maag, Y. Chun, L. Brugger, and M. Grinstein-Weiss. 2022. *The Impacts of the 2021 Expanded Child Tax Credit on Family Employment, Nutrition, and Financial Well-Being*. Available at: https://www.brookings.edu/research/the-impacts-of-the-2021-expanded-child-tax-credit-on-family-employment-nutrition-and-financial-well-being (accessed October 11, 2022).

Held, L. 2022. *Medicaid Is a New Tool to Expand Healthy Food Access*. Available at: https://chlpi.org/news-and-events/news-and-commentary/health-law-and-policy/medicaid-is-a-new-tool-to-expand-healthy-food-access (accessed April 26, 2023).

IOM (Institute of Medicine). 2003. *Unequal Treatment: Confronting Racial and Ethnic Disparities in Health Care*. Washington, DC: The National Academies Press. https://doi.org/10.17226/12875.

IOM. 2014. *Supporting a Movement for Health and Health Equity: Lessons from Social Movements: Workshop Summary*. Washington, DC: The National Academies Press. https://doi.org/10.17226/18751.

Kindig, D. 2022. *The Promise of Population Health: A Scenario for the Next Two Decades*. NAM Perspectives. Commentary. National Academy of Medicine, Washington, DC. https://doi.org/10.31478/202203a.

King, M. W. 2017. Health care efficiencies: Consolidation and alternative models vs. health care and antitrust regulation—Irreconcilable differences? *American Journal of Law & Medicine* 43(4):426-467. https://doi.org/10.1177/0098858817753407.

Leigh, J. P., and J. Du. 2018. *Effects of Minimum Wages on Population Health*. Available at: https://www.healthaffairs.org/do/10.1377/hpb20180622.107025 (accessed February 16, 2023).

Maani, N., and Galea S. 2020. COVID-19 and underinvestment in the public health infrastructure of the United States. *Milbank Quarterly* 98(2):250-259. https://10.1111/1468-0009.12463. Epub 2020 May 13.

Mora, R. D. 2007. *Costa Rica's Commitment: On the Path to Becoming Carbon-Neutral*. Available at: https://www.un.org/en/chronicle/article/costa-ricas-commitment-path-becoming-carbon-neutral (accessed May 11, 2022).

NAM (National Academy of Medicine). 2022. *Emerging Stronger from COVID-19: Priorities for Health System Transformation*. A. Anise, L. Adams, M. Ahmed, A. Bailey, P. S. Chua, C. S. Chukwurah, M. Cocchiola, A. Cupito, K. Kadakia, J.

Lee, and A. Williams, *editors*. NAM Special Publication. Washington, DC: The National Academies Press. https://doi.org/10.17226/26657.

NASI (National Academy of Social Insurance). 2015. *Addressing Pricing Power in Health Care Markets*. Available at: https://www.urban.org/sites/default/files/publication/50116/2000212-Addressing-Pricing-Power-in-Health-Care-Markets.pdf (accessed October 12, 2022).

NIMHD (National Institute on Minority Health and Health Disparities). 2022. *Medicaid Expansion Benefits Young Adults*. Available at: https://www.nimhd.nih.gov/news-events/research-spotlights/medicaid-expansion-benefits-young-adults.html (accessed February 16, 2023).

Nunn, R., J. Parsons, and J. Shambaugh. 2020. *A Dozen Facts About the Economics of the US Health Care System*. Available at: https://www.brookings.edu/research/a-dozen-facts-about-the-economics-of-the-u-s-health-care-system (accessed October 7, 2022).

Office of Senator Chris Murphy. 2022. *Bipartisan Safer Communities Act*. Available at: https://www.murphy.senate.gov/imo/media/doc/bipartisan_safer_communities_act_one_pager.pdf (accessed February 16, 2023).

Peter G. Peterson Foundation. 2022. *U.S. Healthcare System Ranks Sixth Worldwide— Innovative but Fiscally Unsustainable*. Available at: https://www.pgpf.org/blog/2022/01/us-healthcare-system-ranks-sixth-worldwide-innovative-but-fiscally-unsustainable (accessed October 5, 2022).

Shah, T., A. B. Kitts, J. A. Gold, K. Horvath, A. Ommaya, F. Opelka, L. Sato, G. Schwarze, M. Upton, and L. Sandy. 2020. EHR optimization and clinician well-being: A potential roadmap toward action. *NAM Perspectives*. Discussion Paper, National Academy of Medicine, Washington, DC. https://doi.org/10.31478/202008a.

Singletary, K. A., and M. H. Chin. 2023. What should antiracist payment reform look like? *AMA Journal of Ethics* 25(1):E55-E65. https://doi.org/10.1001/amajethics.2023.55.

Tikkanen, R., and M. K. Abrams. 2020. *U.S. Health Care from a Global Perspective, 2019: Higher Spending, Worse Outcomes?* The Commonwealth Fund. Available at: https://www.commonwealthfund.org/publications/issue-briefs/2020/jan/us-health-care-global-perspective-2019 (accessed March 31, 2022).

U.S. Securities and Exchange Commission. 2022. *SEC Proposes to Enhance Disclosures by Certain Investment Advisers and Investment Companies About ESG Investment Practices*. Available at: https://www.sec.gov/news/press-release/2022-92 (accessed October 11, 2022).

Wang, Y., and G. Anderson. 2022. Hospital resource allocation decisions when market prices exceed Medicare prices. *Health Services Research* 57(2):237-247. https://doi.org/10.1111/1475-6773.13914.

Wheatley, M., and D. Frieze. 2006. *Using Emergence to Take Social Innovation to Scale.* Available at: https://margaretwheatley.com/articles/using-emergence.pdf (accessed October 1, 2022).

WHO (World Health Organization). 2022. *Constitution.* Available at: https://www.who.int/about/governance/constitution (accessed June 9, 2022).

Yale University. 2022. *Selling Smoke: Tobacco Advertising and Anti-Smoking Campaigns.* Available at: https://onlineexhibits.library.yale.edu/s/sellingsmoke/page/antismoking (accessed October 4, 2022).

3

PRIORITIZING WHOLE PERSON AND WHOLE POPULATION HEALTH AND WELL-BEING

This section presents illustrative examples of innovative payment and delivery models centered on improving whole person and whole population health and well-being, and that represent key areas of progress aligned with the six key pillars of the Steering Group's vision described in Chapter 2. In doing so, this chapter aims to:

- demonstrate that U.S. health system alignment with whole person and whole population health is achievable;
- provide insight into the core elements essential to the success of innovative models; and
- illustrate the positive health outcomes and savings that payers, providers, individuals, and populations can achieve through a whole person, whole population health approach.

Each of the models described in this section has a unique set of characteristics that can be scaled and replicated across the nation to produce outcomes that are aligned with the six core pillars listed in Box 2. The most critical of these elements are described below. However, it is essential to note that the key factor undergirding each pillar is the prioritization of person-driven supports for health: **empowering individuals to make decisions about their health and well-being within a trusted provider relationship, health care setting, and their communities.**

The Steering Group also derived key lessons from the successes of the models described in the chapter. The following core elements provide the foundation for future efforts to achieve the vision for whole person and whole population health:

1. Aligning financing across payers toward the same goals in a consistent and sustainable way

2. Leadership and structured payment methodologies to incentivize providers and health systems to design and implement multidisciplinary, team-based, and person-driven care to reinforce accountability for whole person and whole population health
3. Addressing the medical and social needs of individuals and populations across the care continuum to achieve equity across different populations
4. Respecting and centering the whole person to consider their culture, family, caregivers, individual needs, preferences, and decisions in the provision of care
5. Improving patient engagement and satisfaction, health outcomes, utilization of health services, and ensuring continuity of care in the design and implementation of health systems
6. Providing services and supports using integrated, innovative, and accessible technology and delivery systems to improve the quality of care through an increased continuum of care, clinical integration, and increased access to services

Although the models described in this chapter do not fully achieve and embody every pillar of the vision as described, they are steps in the right direction. Additionally, each example can act as a case study that engages varying systemic levers to create progress within the present system. Despite the creative attempts and advances in the examples presented below to address systemic issues, they indicate that much progress needs to be made toward whole person and integrative care, which is necessary to address the nation's health crisis.

Key Pillar 1—U.S. health status is at least that of other middle- and high-income countries, with inequities eliminated.

By prioritizing person-centered care, both the Nuka System of Care and the Veterans Health Administration's (VHA's) Whole Health System of Care demonstrate the importance of providing personalized care that addresses patients' concerns, improves health outcomes, and mitigates inequities. The lessons of these models—if more broadly scaled as part of a whole-of-society effort to center whole person, whole population health as the nation's primary goal—would transform health care and public health by focusing on disease prevention, health promotion, and comprehensive care delivery, thereby improving overall health outcomes. Additionally, by incorporating social, environmental, community, and individual factors influencing health, both the Nuka System of Care and the VHA Whole Health System of Care help target the unique and heightened needs of underserved populations and communities nationwide.

SOUTHCENTRAL FOUNDATION'S NUKA SYSTEM OF CARE

Southcentral Foundation's (SCF's) Nuka System of Care, commonly shortened to Nuka, is a whole person–centered health model in Alaska that uses a relationship-based and customer-owned approach to transform health. Nuka provides integrated health services, including medical, dental, behavioral, traditional, and support services to more than 65,000 Alaska Native and American Indian people with a mission of "working together with the Native Community to achieve wellness through health and related services" (Southcentral Foundation, n.d.). The system of care serves 227 federally recognized tribes whose members live in urban, rural, and remote settings across a 108,000-square-mile area (nearly three times the size of Texas).

Implemented following state legislation passed in the late 1990s that allowed Alaska Native populations to take greater control over their health services, Nuka embodies several key features that set it apart from traditional health care models (The King's Fund, n.d.). First, the Alaska Native–owned system emphasizes the community taking ownership of health care, referring to patients as customer-owners. At a system level, customer-owners provide guidance to SCF on system improvement and the development of new programs and services. At an individual and family level, customer-owners drive their health by making informed decisions about health care treatments (Gottlieb et al., 2008). Customer-owners' needs, goals, and values are the system's focus, and they are in control and make decisions rather than a clinician deciding the best treatment. Customer-owner input is routinely solicited through surveys, focus groups, and telephone hotlines (The King's Fund, n.d.).

To ensure the Native community achieves wellness, Nuka uniquely integrates a wide range of professionals in teams providing services such as home and outpatient primary care, dentistry, residential and outpatient behavioral health, traditional healing, integrative medicine, and health education. Across these multidisciplinary care teams, Nuka serves as an administrative conduit that facilitates human resources, information technology, compliance, grants, communications, finance, facility maintenance, and quality management. Cultural recognition and respect are core tenets of this strategy, which is emphasized by appropriate cultural competency training for new employees (Gottlieb, 2013).

In practice, Nuka's management, culture, and technology have removed barriers to quality care for Alaskan communities. The system deploys clinical teams via air or boat to deliver its services in remote areas; utilizes telemedicine to consult on assessment and treatment; and supports the necessary digital infrastructure to collect, aggregate, and share data across care teams to enable complex case management, such as when customer-owners require transportation from a rural community to urban Anchorage for tertiary and specialty services (Gottlieb, 2013).

The outcome improvements behind their numerous awards exemplify the results that a focus on whole person, whole population health can achieve. As of 2013, more than 95 percent of the Alaska Native population was empaneled to an integrated primary care team that understands their histories, preferences, and family context—a stark contrast to the mere 30 percent of the Alaska Native population that had a designated primary care provider in 1996 (Gottlieb, 2013). Additionally, 96 percent of customer-owners reported having input into their care decisions, and 94 percent reported feeling that their culture and traditions are respected (Southcentral Foundation, 2017). More traditional clinical measures of success include:

- Wait times to schedule a routine appointment decreased from 4 weeks to same-day access to a clinician via phone, email, and, if applicable, in-person (Gottlieb, 2013).
- A 40 percent reduction in emergency room visits, 53 percent reduction in hospital admissions, and 65 percent reduction in specialty care usage between 2000 and 2017 due, in large part, to same-day access to care to proactively treat medical conditions before they require more complex care (NIST, 2017).
- 75th-90th percentile rankings for Healthcare Effectiveness Data and Information Set quality measures for diabetes care, cardiovascular LDL, cervical and breast cancer screenings, outpatient and emergency room visits, and pediatric immunization and HPV vaccination rates (Southcentral Foundation, 2017).
- 97 percent of customer-owners and 95 percent of employees reported being satisfied with their experience (*Business Insider*, 2018).

Although the program has been successfully implemented and measured, the diverse funding sources are a challenge to replicate in non-tribal health care settings, where the same mix of funding sources may not overlap. SCF uses key elements of accountable care organizations (ACOs) to operationalize its services, with third party payers such as Medicare, Medicaid, and some private insurers providing approximately 48 percent of its operating revenue (Salinsky, 2017; Southcentral Foundation, n.d.). The federal Indian Health Service makes up the majority of the remainder, providing approximately 45 percent through a payment mechanism similar to a block grant that is not based on the volume of services (Salinsky, 2017). The remaining 5 percent comes from grants and 2 percent from investment and other sources (Salinsky, 2017).

Nevertheless, this model exemplifies the benefits of a relentless focus on individual experience and centricity—from cost savings to health outcomes and overall well-being (Salinsky, 2017). The model's outcomes also demonstrate the benefits of transforming systems; the Nuka System of Care realigned financial incentives toward prioritizing access to primary care and a wide continuum of services and supports such as behavioral health services. A cultural transformation was also implemented, with patients recognized as "customer-owners" with unique experiences, contexts, and preferences (Salinsky, 2017).

VETERANS HEALTH ADMINISTRATION'S WHOLE HEALTH SYSTEM OF CARE

The VHA funds and promotes the Whole Health System of Care (WHS), an advanced form of patient-centered care that empowers veterans to become engaged in their own health and well-being. The approach shifts the traditional conversation with each patient from "What is the matter with you?" to "What matters *to* you?" (Bokhour et al., 2020a). Complemented by a robust online resource and information center, veterans engaged in the WHS establish their own personal health plan based on a personal health inventory created via self-assessment. This allows veterans to create individualized sets of services and supports based on what matters most to the individual (VA, 2022).

A central feature of creating the personal health plan involves veterans considering the VA Circle of Health, which illustrates the connections between an individual, their clinical health, their well-being, and the healing relationships, environment, and community that surrounds each aspect (see Figure 3). This tool can be used to help individuals to determine their current position relative to their health, their personal goals, the actions they can take, and the interventions that can help them achieve their goals (VA, 2021).

In the WHS program, allopathic medicine and behavioral medicine are combined with an integrative set of health interventions, each structured to meet the priorities and goals of individual patients. Key services at the core of WHS include:

- Personalized health planning helps individuals to identify the health foci most important to their own personal goals;
- Peer-led whole health courses build a community of veterans working toward whole health; and
- Whole Health Pathway services, well-being programs, and coaching to support veterans working to achieve their whole health goals.

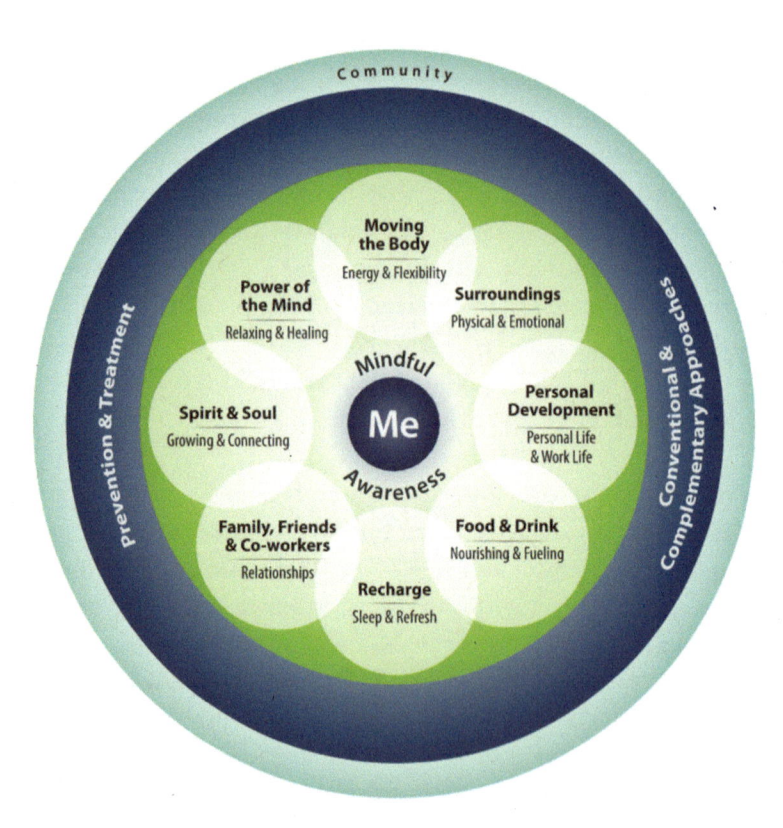

FIGURE 3 | U.S. Veterans Health Administration Circle of Health.
SOURCE: VA, 2021.

Veterans engaged in WHS are encouraged to explore complementary services as well, including chiropractic care, massage, acupuncture, yoga, tai chi, meditation, guided imagery, biofeedback, and hypnosis as possible ways to exercise, reduce stress, and recover from injuries.

Access to WHS services is provided through online resources such as telehealth and a robust set of digital resources that have been in place since before the COVID-19 pandemic. In 2019, more than 10,000 complementary and integrative health visits were had among almost 4,000 veterans, a four-fold increase in usage since 2018 (Whitehead and Kligler, 2020). In response to the COVID-19 pandemic, the utility of this approach was fully realized and implemented, with WHS sites using telehealth to conduct patient wellness calls and institute self-care strategies, complementary and integrative health therapies, and stress-management tools for providers and patients alike. The utility of these strategies for staff as well as veterans was a key tool to combat the clinician burnout that has accompanied the many tragedies of the COVID-19 pandemic. In doing so, it allowed for a healthier, more resilient workforce, empowered to provide for the individuals they serve (Reddy et al., 2021).

In 2018, the VHA launched 18 Whole Health Flagship facilities to evaluate WHS and to examine utilization data and health outcomes. In sites in which WHS was implemented, 31 percent of veterans suffering from chronic pain engaged in one or more Whole Health pain services. At one site, 55 percent of veterans with chronic pain were reported to have used at least one Whole Health service. From 2017 to 2019, utilization by veterans of Whole Health services grew across VA sites, including a 193 percent increase in utilization among veterans with chronic pain, a 211 percent increase among those with mental health diagnoses, and a 272 percent increase among those with chronic conditions (see Table 1). During these years, the use of complementary or integrative health services more than doubled (Bokhour et al., 2020b).

This increase in utilization seems to have had a positive impact on participating veterans. Studies have demonstrated that opioid use decreased among Whole Health users, dependent on their level of engagement with Whole Health services. Among veterans with chronic pain who used Whole Health services, opioid use declined by up to 38 percent, a three-fold greater reduction than the 11 percent decline in opioid use by veterans who did not use Whole Health (Bokhour et al., 2020b).

Other preliminary data from these flagship sites revealed that, compared to non-participating veterans, individuals who participated in Whole Health services reported greater improvements in perceptions of care, engagement in health care, self-care, life meaning and purpose, pain reduction, and perceived stress. Preliminary research compiled in 2019 from the Flagship sites is being studied to estimate the impact of the program on health care costs, although data from 2018 indicate an estimated 24 percent drop in total health care costs among participating veterans, particularly surrounding pharmacy costs (Bokhour et al., 2020b).

The successes of the Nuka System of Care and the VHA's Whole System of Care—both in terms of traditional process and outcomes measures as well as patient-defined indicators of success—provide key learnings to realizing a nationwide vision of whole person, whole population health. The Nuka System of Care involves significant buy-in from organizational leadership, employees, and customers in delivering and accepting transformational change and a realignment of resources and services (Salinsky, 2017). These drivers of success, if scaled nationally, have the potential to unlock widespread health and well-being if stakeholder priorities, resources, and actions are aligned. To implement these changes, as exemplified by the VHA's Whole System of Care, personalized health planning with the engagement, trust, and voice of patients is required. The power

TABLE 1 | Whole Health Service Use Among Veterans with Chronic Pain, Mental Health Diagnoses, and Chronic Conditions from the First Quarter of 2017 to the Third Quarter of 2019*

	Veterans with Chronic Pain			Veterans with a Mental Health Diagnosis			Veterans with Chronic Conditions		
	Q1FY17	Q3FY19	% Change	Q1FY17	Q3FY19	% Change	Q1FY17	Q3FY19	% Change
Any Whole Health System Service	10.5%	30.7%	193%	7.4%	23.2%	211%	4.4%	16.4%	272%
Any Complementary or Integrative Service	10.3%	26.4%	158%	7.2%	19.3%	169%	4.2%	12.8%	206%

* The identified sample includes 114,357 veterans with chronic pain; 149,621 veterans with anxiety, depression, and post-traumatic stress disorder (PTSD); and 229,646 veterans with a common chronic condition. The groups are overlapping.
SOURCE: Bokhour et al., 2020b.

of science and medicine must also be combined with the lived realities, context, and complexities of all individuals who access and receive care.

Key Pillar 2—Health and health equity are nationwide commitments spanning beyond organizations in health care and public health.

Improving the health of populations, communities, and individuals requires a whole-of-society approach in which all actors, including those outside of the traditional domains of health care and public health, prioritize health and health equity. Adventist Health's Blue Zones, employer-based worksite wellness programs, and school-based health centers exemplify the need to prioritize health in the critical and impactful settings of work, school, and the community at large.

ADVENTIST HEALTH'S BLUE ZONES

Acquired by Adventist Health in 2020, Blue Zones takes a systems-focused and community-based approach to improving well-being at the population level. The organization provides consulting, convening, and implementation services that help strengthen population-level health and well-being. For example, instead of aiming to change individual behavior (e.g., urging people to diet and exercise), the Blue Zones Life Radius model focuses on making healthy choices the default (i.e., easier) in all the places where individuals spend the most time—where they live, work, learn, play, and pray. By making lasting changes to the human-made surroundings and systems that determine health and life outcomes, people are collectively nudged to move and connect more, eat better, and develop a healthy outlook as they move throughout their day.

Rather than a siloed approach that concentrates on specific health challenges, Blue Zones represents a paradigm shift that focuses on root causes. This recognition of the built environment that individuals live within has been shown to be sustainable, increasing dividends for future residents. Examples of optimizing the built environment to improve community well-being include improving roads and transportation options, parks, and public spaces and building healthier options in the places people spend most of their time, such as restaurants, schools, and grocery stores. Additional Blue Zones interventions include building indoor sports arenas, expanding community garden space, increasing walking times to school, and restricting tobacco use.

These community initiatives are public-private partnerships, with the majority of funding typically sourced from a singular private entity (e.g., health care systems, health insurers, health organizations, or a coalition of entities). A major driver of funding is the notion that people with higher measures of well-being live a fuller life in which they can contribute to their community without the financial hardships that often accompany acute health care costs. Simply put, optimizing well-being is in the best interest of the vast majority of actors within a community and, as such, community partners and sponsors have often come together to empower Blue Zones, as they have been shown to reduce the burden of lower well-being and chronic disease on their neighbors, local economies, health care systems, and productivity. Participating communities have seen double-digit reductions in obesity and smoking and significant improvements in health risks and productivity (IOM, 2015).

The implementation of the Blue Zones model in Albert Lea, Minnesota, for example, was associated with a 40 percent reduction in health care costs for city workers, 2.9 years added to life spans within 1 year of participation, a collective weight loss of 7,280 pounds, and a downtown streetscape revitalization that has increased private investment, tourism, and the community's tax base (Blue Zones, 2022a). Since Blue Zone programs were implemented in Fort Worth, Texas, in 2014, the city moved from the 185th healthiest city in the nation to the 31st healthiest city in the nation (Blue Zones, 2022b). Neighborhoods and sectors of Fort Worth with citizens who exhibited the highest well-being disparities in 2014 also showed gains in well-being as of 2022: a major bright spot at a time when higher risk populations disparately experience poorer health outcomes and higher health care costs (Blue Zones, 2022b).

EMPLOYER-BASED WORKSITE WELLNESS PROGRAMS

American employers are the largest providers of health coverage in the United States, serving approximately 163 million workers and their families through private-sector employment-based plans (Mattke et al., 2015). These employers are witnessing rising rates of diabetes, obesity, and heart disease, among other chronic conditions, many of which are driven by social determinants of health (SDoH) and unhealthy behaviors such as smoking, excessive alcohol use, poor nutrition, and inactivity (Mattke et al., 2015). These chronic conditions are among the costliest to treat and often lead to a lower quality of life, higher health care costs, early-onset disability, and premature death. Therefore, in a national sector-wide transformation, employer-based health programs can contribute to improved whole health.

It is clearly in the best interest of employers to invest in employee well-being, especially when faced with the stark reality of annual per capita costs associated with health risks. High employee blood glucose is associated with a $129 increase in per capita costs; stress is associated with a $118 increase in per capita costs; depression is associated with a $71 increase in per capita costs; and physical inactivity is associated with an $82 increase in per capita costs (Goetzel et al., 2020). Since 2019 the cost to employers for employees' mental disorders alone equals more than $200 billion annually—mostly in lost productivity (Goetzel et al., 2018).

As major health care payers, it benefits employers to find innovative solutions that address ever-rising health and health care costs (Blumenthal et al., 2018). Additionally, given that most Americans work full-time jobs, a major opportunity exists to promote health and wellness in the context of the work setting and the social networks it provides. Through a creative redesign of traditional corporate and organizational care delivery and wellness programs, work settings can further empower individuals to make healthy lifestyle changes by creating environments, programs, practices, expectations, and habits that naturally move people toward healthier choices. Large-scale interventions include paying all employees a living wage, re-evaluating sick leave policies to maximize their use, and sliding scale health insurance premiums based on income. More frequently embraced small-scale interventions include onsite smoking bans, healthy food choices, and socially connective groups such as workplace book clubs, cooking classes, or exercise programs. Employers can build on these approaches by linking provider incentives with employee incentives so the two parties work toward common goals. To address transportation and child care costs, decrease carbon emissions, as well as improve worker well-being, employers could also consider hybrid and/or remote work policies that maintain social cohesion and organizational performance.

The goal of worksite health promotion programs focusing on the root causes of poor health is to reduce the need for avoidable care and medications and to enhance employee well-being. These programs offer a convenient, supportive venue for employees to learn about healthier lifestyles that can prevent, treat, and reverse disease and embrace the broader construct of whole person and whole population health. As an example, employers such as Cummins, Inc., an American multinational corporation that designs, manufactures, and distributes power generation products, has included integrative and complementary practices in their onsite clinics. In their largest clinic located in Columbus, Indiana, Cummins, Inc., successfully integrated chiropractic, acupuncture, and therapeutic massage with traditional physical therapy and orthopedic referrals for the care and treatment of musculoskeletal conditions.

Another company, Statistical Analysis System (SAS), has extensive health care and wellness programs, including onsite health care with free physician appointments that encourage workers to seek treatment for physical and mental health as soon as needed. Colocation of physicians at the worksite reduces travel time to doctors' offices, helping employees overcome locational barriers to access. An evaluation of SAS's wellness offerings found that each dollar spent on the onsite clinic saves $2.24, producing $6.6 billion in annual savings and supporting 96 percent worker retention (Sholl, n.d.). While these findings are promising, it is important to recognize that common methodological challenges, such as lack of a control group and a short-term pre- versus post-analyses, render many evaluations of this type more suggestive than probative.

SCHOOL-BASED HEALTH CENTERS

A significant amount of care for children is provided in or through schools and is often paid for by Medicaid. This offers an innovative opportunity—both for integrated health service delivery and flexible financing—that is supportive of the vision described throughout this publication (MACPAC, 2018). In fiscal year (FY) 2016, Medicaid covered more than 4.5 billion for school-based care and related administrative services provided to students that meet certain criteria (MACPAC, 2018). School-based health centers (SBHCs) leverage this funding as a key driver of community-wide pediatric health, providing students with a single point of access for trustworthy, person-centered, culturally informed, and integrated care across multiple colocated providers. These centers have been found to improve educational outcomes, including school performance, grade promotion, and high school completion, while also improving health outcomes, including the delivery of vaccinations and other recommended preventive services, decreasing asthma morbidity, and decreasing emergency department use and hospital admission (Community Preventive Services Task Force, 2015).

Key examples of these vast and varied health centers include New York City's (NYC's) SBHCs within roughly 387 schools that help students manage their health needs throughout the school day. Such care centers have provided primary care for more than 25 years, lowering school absences and decreasing parents' time away from work (NYC DOE, 2022). The centers are run by local hospitals, medical centers, and community organizations and are overseen by the New York State Department of Health and the NYC Department of Health and Mental Hygiene. They provide care regardless of insurance status but remain funded through Medicaid and private insurance billing, where applicable.

SBHCs have also demonstrated positive impact in underserved rural areas. In Montana, the Assiniboine and Sioux Tribes of the Fort Peck Reservation experience high rates of poverty, life expectancy more than 20 years lower than the state average, 50 percent unemployment, and a less than 70 percent high school graduation rate (Harvard Project, 2015). Tribal youth experience higher rates of smoking, alcohol use, exposure to violence, trauma, and suicide. Almost 50 percent of children attending the reservation's schools are overweight or obese, and more than 60 percent have untreated tooth decay (Harvard Project, 2015). In response to these challenges, the tribes created a SBHC initiative to offer integrated services for their children in schools, employing evidence-based medicine in concert with the local culture and traditions of the tribes. The centers serve more than 1,100 children, with participation varying across centers from 75 percent to 95 percent of enrolled students, and are primarily funded by Medicaid reimbursement (Harvard Project, 2015).

Depending on their design and implementation, there is strong evidence that SBHCs generate myriad benefits (County Health Rankings & Roadmaps, 2023). By increasing access to care, including immunization, nutritional, physical activity, and screening services, SBHCs can reduce emergency room visits and hospital utilization; prevent sexually transmitted infections, teen pregnancies, and substance abuse; improve mental health; and enhance educational outcomes (County Health Rankings & Roadmaps, 2023). These impacts, especially when applied in a culturally competent manner in historically or presently marginalized communities, offer a key opportunity to reduce systemic discrimination and health care access gaps across race, geographic location, sexual orientation and gender identity, income, and disability status (County Health Rankings & Roadmaps, 2023).

Despite documented successes, it is important to note that attaining the full promise of integrated health and community services within and aligned with schools remains a challenge. While for many children, schools are a center for education, nutrition, and food security, the limited number of SBHCs nationwide leaves many children without access to these services. Creative use of blended and braided funding models, increased coverage of services delivered in schools by Medicaid and private insurers, a more robust school health workforce, and community support of care within schools can translate to a fully realized potential of better education and health outcomes for many school-aged children.

Despite operating under the above-mentioned constraints, Adventist Health's Blue Zones, employer-based workplace wellness sites, and SBHCs demonstrate the ability to promote whole person, whole population health without the leadership of the traditional health care and public health ecosystem. By targeting the myriad of influences, factors, and drivers of health where people live, work, and learn, these and other efforts to reform social, behavioral, and environmental infrastructure at the local level; comprehensively support employee health and well-being; and pool state and national funds to promote student health are integral to equitably improving the nation's health.

Key Pillar 3—Health care expenditures as a percentage of gross domestic product (GDP) do not constrain and displace other important social services that directly impact health and equity.

Current U.S. health care expenditures far exceed the norm for peer countries globally, especially when considered alongside a set of population-level health outcomes that are worse relative to comparable nations. While aligning resources and incentives with innovative care is a major priority for health system transformation, the scope of these efforts should be widened to reduce health care expenditures to a percentage of GDP that better aligns with Organisation of Economic Co-operation and Development (OECD) benchmarks. By introducing cost containment strategies, barriers to accessing care are reduced and care delivery organizations would be compelled to innovate to provide better care quality. The state of Maryland provides an excellent case study on how to reduce health care costs in a way that fosters high-quality care.

MARYLAND ALL-PAYER AND TOTAL COST OF CARE MODEL

Maryland's unique all-payer model aims to promote the health and well-being of state residents while controlling the cost of health care. This model is based on a hospital rate-setting system that dates back to the 1970s, during which an independent Health Services Cost Review Commission set fee-for-service rates for each hospital that applied to all of the hospital's payers, including the uninsured (Jain et al., 2022). A provision in the Social Security Act permitted Medicare to participate in Maryland's program and, as other states abandoned rate-setting efforts in the 1980s, Maryland opted to continue. This approach led to slower growth in the hospital rates charged in Maryland than in the rest of the country (Murray, 2009).

Maryland's historic experience prepared the state for change in 2014. By this time, it had become clear that fee-for-service rate-setting had limits; for example, while rate growth had been limited, volume growth had not been constrained. After extensive discussions within the state and with federal regulators, the Center for Medicare & Medicaid Innovation (CMMI) approved a new iteration of the Maryland Model in 2014. This reform fundamentally changed the state's approach to hospital payment in that it required the Health Services Cost Review Commission to set prospective global budgets for hospitals. Generally speaking, these budgets would cover hospital inpatient and outpatient charges, regardless of patient volume, and rate-setting mechanisms would be used to help hospitals receive the revenue set by their global budgets from payers.

As the new Maryland Model was implemented, the financial incentives facing hospitals changed dramatically. Previously, under fee-for-service rate-setting, preventing hospitalizations attributed fixed costs to each hospital's bottom line. With global budgets, however, preventing hospitalizations could be financially advantageous, as the hospital's revenue would be unaffected. Hospitals across Maryland began to invest in a wide range of programs to keep patients from needing hospital care.

An independent evaluation from RTI International found that the Maryland Model led to major changes in care delivery, including a range of partnerships to support care coordination and transitions, as well as the fact that "nearly all hospitals invested in care coordination, discharge planning, social work staffing, patient care transition plans, and systematic use of patient care plans in response to the All-Payer model" (RTI, 2019). In terms of costs, RTI found the Maryland Model to be associated with a 2.8 percent decline in Medicare expenditures (including a 4.1 percent decline in hospital expenditures) without cost shifting elsewhere (RTI, 2019). This represented Medicare savings of about $1 billion. There were also substantial and statistically significant reductions in all hospital admissions and potentially avoidable hospital admissions for Medicare beneficiaries, and evidence of benefits to commercial payers (RTI, 2019).

In 2019, the state updated the Maryland Model, agreeing to a new 8-year arrangement with CMMI (Sapra et al., 2019). The new version, termed the Total Cost of Care model, added a primary care program to support care transformation and a care redesign program to allow hospitals to make incentive payments to specialist providers and suppliers; it also facilitated investments in outpatient and crisis behavioral health services and added more explicit expectations for reductions in the Medicare total cost of care (to total $2 billion in savings over the 8-year period) (Machta et al., 2021). In the first year, Maryland generated $365 million in Medicare savings. The state has also set population health goals for diabetes, addiction and overdose, childhood asthma, and maternal mortality (Machta et al., 2021).

The statewide scale of Maryland's model and its initial successes are unique in the health policy landscape, but several concepts are inspiring others to apply and scale it to their own jurisdictions. Pennsylvania has expanded global budgeting to rural hospitals, and through the Community Health Access and Rural Transformation (CHART) model, CMMI may allow other rural hospitals to follow a similar path. Even as the state attracts more attention, the model is still a work in progress. Key efforts include producing more cost savings, creating more capacity and support for behavioral health care, closer community-hospital connections, and more ambitious population health efforts.

Health care models that promote cost savings while delivering high-quality care and optimal outcomes at scale remain an elusive goal. As the nation experiences successive health crises, there is a pressing need to expand involvement beyond the health care system. While transforming the health care system will impact 15-20 percent of the U.S. economy, there should also be clear economic and cultural incentives that encourage health-promoting actions and investments across the U.S. economy.

Key Pillar 4—Economic and cultural incentives encourage every stakeholder sector to take health promoting actions and make health promoting investments.

Aligned financing mechanisms help reinforce accountability for whole person and whole population health outcomes. This section describes programs and models that exemplify the concept of sustainable incentives for health improvement, including the Healthy Neighborhoods Equity Fund and Third-Party Investor Collaboration in Community Wellness. The section also describes the experience of the Casey Health Institute, which, despite its innovative vision, was stymied by an unhelpful payment structure.

HEALTHY NEIGHBORHOODS EQUITY FUND

Healthy Neighborhoods Equity Fund II (HNEF II) is an innovative $50 million private equity real estate fund that addresses the SDoH by investing in community-responsive development intended to:

1. expand housing choice and affordability;
2. provide access to transit, jobs, green space, and healthy food;
3. support local wealth creation; and
4. increase resilience to climate change (Church and Flatley, 2020; HNEF, 2022a).

The fund is cosponsored by Conservation Law Foundation (CLF), a nonprofit environmental advocacy organization, and Massachusetts Housing Investment Corporation, a community development financial institution (CDFI). HNEF II supports high-impact development in historically disinvested communities that are experiencing significant health and economic disparities, as well as opportunity-rich communities with excellent public schools where the fund can help deepen affordability for families with children. The fund, which operates in Massachusetts, Connecticut, and Rhode Island, fills a critical financing gap by providing lower-cost, longer-term equity capital that is otherwise unavailable in the market. HNEF II pools funding from multiple institutional and individual investors, including hospitals, health plans, banks, and high net worth individuals to make these investments possible.

To ensure that HNEF investments achieve meaningful health and community impacts, all development projects are screened through HealthScore—a comprehensive impact scorecard developed and managed by CLF. HealthScore is a holistic, place-based, context-specific assessment tool that integrates both quantitative and qualitative measures in order to understand the need, opportunity, and likelihood of impact across multiple domains, such as housing affordability, job creation, walkability, climate resilience, and energy efficiency (CLF, 2021). Importantly, the fund only invests in development that has strong community support and has demonstrated responsiveness to the needs and priorities of local residents. In total, HealthScore includes more than 100 objective measures that help inform and support investment decision-making while also providing guidance to developers about what they can do to maximize health benefits for residents (CLF, 2021). To be considered for an HNEF investment, development proposals must receive a minimum score of 50 out of 100; developments that score higher receive more favorable consideration (HNEF, 2022b). HealthScore was originally created in 2014 for Healthy Neighborhoods Equity Fund I and is based on two health impact assessments conducted by the Metropolitan Area Planning Council as well as findings from the Healthy Neighborhoods Study (HNS), a longitudinal Participatory Action Research study conducted by CLF in partnership with the Massachusetts Institute of Technology, nine community-based organizations, and more than 40 resident researchers (Larson, 2021). HNEF's use of HealthScore to screen and score investments has been a particularly important aspect of the fund for health care investors seeking to use their financial assets to improve the health of communities beyond the provision of acute clinical care (Church, 2018).

As neighborhoods across the country grapple with the combined impacts of housing and health crises exacerbated by COVID-19 and worsened by climate change, it is even more imperative that the health care sector be an active participant in long-term, sustainable solutions. HNEF provides a platform for health care to invest in healthier, more inclusive, and more resilient neighborhoods in a way that benefits the individuals who need them the most (Church and McGilvray, 2018). Before HNEF I investments, existing residents in the selected neighborhoods were 50 percent more likely to be admitted to the hospital for diabetes, and nearly 57 percent were housing cost-burdened, constraining their ability to afford other basic necessities (HNEF, 2020). In response to these and other challenges, HNEF I and II have supported the creation of 688 new mixed-income homes to date, including both rental units and those that are now owned outright, that are affordable to households earning between 30 percent and 110 percent of Area Median Income (HNEF, 2020; UnitedHealth Group, 2022).

HNEF I and II investments have also supported the creation of more than 139,000 square feet of commercial space, enabling local entrepreneurs to open new health-promoting businesses, including healthy food outlets and gyms that cater to residents of the surrounding neighborhood (HNEF, 2022a). Additionally, the fund cosponsors have committed to addressing the racial wealth gap by ensuring that the benefits of their investments flow to local workers, including workers of color that are often left out of large construction contracts or have been hurt most by COVID-19 (Dana-Farber Cancer Institute, 2021). For every dollar of HNEF I investment, 91 cents went to Minority Business Enterprises (MBEs); in total, HNEF I supported nearly $20 million in MBE construction contract volume. These types of upstream investments in the SDoH are particularly important for communities that have been disinvested over generations, many of which are now experiencing the additional stressors of gentrification and displacement (Binet et al., 2021). Responding to these structural challenges through place-based and people-centered investment is essential to population health improvement. Health care is an essential partner in this work.

CHI HEALTH CARE/THE CASEY HEALTH INSTITUTE

In 2012, CHI Health Care (formerly the Casey Health Institute) piloted a grant-funded, public, nonprofit integrative primary care community health center in Gaithersburg, Maryland. CHI Health Care was an early adopter of the patient-centered medical home framework with a clinical team that included an interdisciplinary staff combining conventional primary care with a wide array of natural and complementary healing disciplines and integrative health. Team collaboration was emphasized through regular weekly meetings, electronic communication avenues, and informal interactions. The staff of practitioners included family medicine, internal medicine, integrative medicine, naturopathic medicine, acupuncture, traditional Chinese medicine, chiropractic care, psychology, psychotherapy, mindfulness, behavioral health, nutrition, yoga therapy, health coaching, therapeutic massage, and extensive health, wellness, and lifestyle medicine programming.

CHI increased access to high-quality, cost-effective health care across community members spanning the socioeconomic spectrum by accepting commercial health insurance, Medicare and Medicaid, and offering a sliding scale for the uninsured and underinsured. CHI allocated the resources necessary to build the infrastructure to transition from fee-for-service reimbursement to value-based care and population health payment models. It participated in initiatives such as the Centers for Medicare & Medicaid Services' (CMS's) Medicare Shared Savings Plan and the CareFirst patient-centered medical home (PCMH) incentive program, thereby increasing access to CHI Health Care's services and supports.

CHI was founded on the principle of embracing payment models that incentivized primary care while discouraging the overuse of invasive procedures and unnecessary treatments. It focused resources on health information technology through a robust patient portal, telemedicine with video medical appointments, electronic health record data tracking, outcomes research, team member electronic collaboration, and care coordination by capturing real-time data from the Maryland state health information exchange. The data CHI collected during its 6-year pilot demonstrated that 95 percent of patients were highly satisfied with their care and experienced fewer urgent care services, less prescription medication, and lower hospital admissions and readmission rates compared to patients of comparable conventional practices.

CHI Health Care succeeded in significantly improving health outcomes with lower downstream costs and consistently high levels of patient and staff satisfaction. However, the project ultimately failed because key population health infrastructure, care coordination, and essential health and wellness professional staff were not adequately compensated by either the existing fee-for-service environment or the value-based payment platforms available in Maryland at that time. CHI's business plan was based on the projection that by rewarding value and not volume, value-based care programs would become more widely available and the incentives rewarding such practices would increase over time in the form of higher rates.

HNEFs I and II succeeded due to their ability to balance a respectable return on investment while investing in infrastructure to improve housing affordability and encourage MBEs. Meanwhile, CHI Health Care's failure exposes the difficulties for providers to remain competitive in a landscape dominated by fee-for-service payment. While CHI generated value for their patients, the process of rewarding value over volume remains highly challenging. In the current payment environment, a few key insights might make a similar model successful today. These key facilitators include:

- Appropriately compensated collaborative interdisciplinary team care is an essential part of a comprehensive whole person health care system. This team includes all levels of primary care clinicians, practice support staff (including care coordination and population health positions), and a broad representation of integrative health professionals.

- A salaried staff model with a non-hierarchical organizational structure that facilitates essential ongoing collaboration is critical for success.
- Economies of scale are necessary. Optimal health creation and preservation in a primary care environment is expensive if implemented in a free-standing community-based practice. Shared resources for practice administration, human resources, information technology, medical supplies, and salaried personnel are needed across practices to provide negotiating power to capture optimal value-based contracts.
- An end goal of negotiated capitated contracts with two-sided risk on a per member, per month basis. This goal would ensure that CHI would not only share in care savings but also be held accountable for spending above cost benchmarks. Value-based payments based on this structure would allow for the best and sustainable use of a collaborative, interdisciplinary team model.

THIRD-PARTY INVESTOR COLLABORATION IN COMMUNITY WELLNESS

Social impact investing has increased in recent decades, along with three broad phenomena:

- Growing wealth and income inequality, which also created large classes of investors looking to do good while earning acceptable returns;
- Declining trust in government and corresponding strains on the capacity to meet underserved communities' basic needs; and
- Increasing evidence that solutions exist for common problems but financing at scale is precluded by current law or traditional capital market failures.

The U.S. Impact Investing Alliance identifies several sources of community investments and financing, including corporations, Community Reinvestment Act–motivated banks, CDFIs, foundations and family offices, high-net-worth individuals, fintech[1]/crowdfunding, and community-investing participation models (U.S. Impact Investing Alliance, 2021). For example, corporations such as PayPal and the Black Economic Development Fund by Local Initiatives Support Coalition (LISC) provided deposits and other support to Black-owned banks in response to calls for racial justice (U.S. Impact Investing Alliance, 2021). The Grow with Google Small Business Fund supports the financing needs of small

---

[1] Fintech refers to financial technology and describes "new tech that seeks to improve and automate the delivery and use of financial services"; see https://www.investopedia.com/terms/f/fintech.asp (accessed September 29, 2022).

businesses in distressed communities (U.S. Impact Investing Alliance, 2021). The Ujima Fund is a participatory model for local restorative wealth building and small dollar investor engagement (U.S. Impact Investing Alliance, 2021).

Place-based investments, traditionally in the realm of CDFIs, have been arranged by increasingly entrepreneurial health anchor institutions, such as Intermountain Healthcare, which has created a self-sustaining fund from its community benefit dollars that makes loans and investments to local community-based organizations (CBOs) to address a range of SDoH needs, including affordable housing, rural community development, and complex case management (Build Healthy Places Network, 2021). The Healthcare Anchor Network is an umbrella group with 70 health systems that are doing similar work to Intermountain Health across the country (Healthcare Anchor Network, 2022). Additionally, Quantified Ventures, an investment and consulting firm, designs a continuum of outcomes-based financing approaches for SDoH by aligning CBOs and impact investors on a set of outcomes that are valued by all. Impact investors deliver flexible capital to build capacity and scale services to more people, CBOs focus on improving outcomes through service delivery, and payers ultimately repay investors if and when pre-specified outcomes are achieved. Investors secure both a social and financial return on their investment if project outcomes are achieved. Recent examples of their work in SDoH include food delivery, medical respite for patients experiencing homelessness, and substance use treatment and prevention for prospective moms and babies (Quantified Ventures, 2021a,b,c).

Key Pillar 5—Efforts from all sectors, including government programs and regulations, are organized to prioritize the health of individuals, communities, and society.

Designing public and private programs and services to maximize the health of individuals and communities can help to ensure that the most underserved members of society have equitable access to economic and social support interventions. Initiatives such as the Program of All-Inclusive Care for the Elderly, Medicare Advantage Special Needs Plans, and Medicaid Long Term Services and Supports are effective examples of this concept in action.

PROGRAM OF ALL-INCLUSIVE CARE FOR THE ELDERLY

The Program of All-Inclusive Care for the Elderly (PACE) model of care is built on the belief that community-based whole person care is better for the well-being of seniors with chronic care needs, as well as their families and caregivers

(PACE, 2022). This integrated model of care serves individuals 55 or older who meet nursing home level of care requirements and are able to live safely in the community. PACE provides the entire continuum of care and services, including medical care and support services such as adult day care, transportation, laundry support, meals, nutritional counseling, social services, home health care, personal care, and respite care. Unlike many other models of care, a fundamental requirement in PACE is a coordinated, cross-sector interdisciplinary team of providers. This team includes drivers, personal care attendants, recreational therapists, and activity directors who collaborate with primary care physicians, nurses, and social workers who convene regularly to discuss patient care needs.

PACE is a statutorily combined Medicare and Medicaid payment and delivery system model that is designed specifically to enhance whole person care in the community. The program's unique status as a model authorized directly by federal statute is critical to its success as an integrated, whole person model. Its permanent statutory authorization guarantees a clear, consistent, and sustained financing source within Medicare and Medicaid and a transparent methodology that allows providers to make long-term investments. The PACE statute also specifies Medicare and Medicaid benefits and eligible provider types, providing clarity and sustainability for both in the financing methodologies. Taken together, the three statutorily defined aspects of PACE—financing, benefits, and provider types—are intertwined into one sustainable care model.

As of July 2021, PACE has expanded across 30 states. More than 270 PACE centers provide services to 55,000 seniors, 95 percent of whom live in their communities (PACE, 2020). The program is primarily financed through a prospective risk-adjusted monthly capitated payment methodology (CMS, 2011). The vast majority (90 percent) of PACE members are dual-eligible enrollees, who are individuals enrolled in both Medicare and Medicaid. Nine percent of remaining PACE members are covered through Medicaid only, while 1 percent are either covered by Medicare or through other means. Medicare-only enrollees pay monthly premiums equal to the Medicaid capitation amount and do not pay deductibles, coinsurance, or any other cost-sharing (CMS, n.d.-a).

Despite the fact that PACE participants experience fewer emergency department visits, reduced hospital admissions and readmissions, and lower costs of care (PACE, 2020), the program continues to struggle with scaling to the much larger population of potential beneficiaries. Barriers to wider dissemination include:

- high start-up and expansion costs for providers;
- the unwillingness of potential beneficiaries to change physicians, plans, or residential facilities or to attend adult day centers;

- the resource-intensiveness of care planning and coordination;
- the current narrowly defined beneficiary population that is eligible to participate;
- lack of flexibility within the model to tailor benefits packages and financing; and
- high costs for regulatory compliance (Thomson Reuters, 2011).

Strides toward greater uptake of the model could be made through additional action by Congress to address these concerns or by requiring CMS to test the expansion of a model similar to PACE in additional populations, such as for pregnant women in Medicaid, CHIP, or for individuals with intellectual or developmental disabilities, regardless of age.

The struggle to scale PACE surfaces issues around long-term funding of future care models as well as the disconnected statutory authority of CMS and the Social Security Administration in creating and disseminating comprehensively integrated care models. First, while innovative care models, such as those developed and implemented by CMMI, provide an opportunity to test integrated benefit design and payment methodologies across funding streams, they carry greater uncertainty with respect to the availability of future funding. By law, the sustainability of each CMMI model is dependent on its own success and future decisions by policy makers. The lack of guaranteed long-term Medicare and Medicaid financing acts as a deterrent for larger-scale disruption to create integrated care models as well as for investment in such models. Because these models necessarily carry more risk, they are less attractive to providers, who would be required to implement disruptive innovations to improve care and outcomes within the relatively short 2- to 5-year time frame of a model. Additionally, without the guarantee of statutorily protected blended financing across Medicare and Medicaid, states, health plans, and providers have, in large part, lacked sufficient incentives to overcome rational risk aversion.

Second, there is limited legal authority to create and implement models similar to PACE. PACE is unique as the PACE statute allows the program to go beyond the limits of CMMI's statute as a key provision of the Affordable Care Act as well as the authority of section 1115A of the Social Security Act. As a Medicare program, PACE can be provided to Medicaid beneficiaries should states elect to provide PACE services to Medicaid beneficiaries (Medicaid, n.d.).

Limited waiver authority makes it challenging to craft truly integrated models or to innovate whole-person care models. As a result of this limited waiver authority, Medicare and Medicaid cannot be synced or permitted by law unless Medicare aligns with the Medicaid statute. In comparison, the PACE statutory language in

Medicaid exactly mirrors that of Medicare, creating a fully integrated program across the two funding streams—such that the same definitions and specifications for benefits, providers, and payment apply. Therefore, policy makers should clarify the legal authority of Medicare, Medicaid, and the Social Security Administration so that these programs can build more coherent and complementary policies that promote whole health.

MEDICARE ADVANTAGE SPECIAL NEEDS PLANS

The Medicare Modernization Act of 2003 (MMA) established Medicare Advantage Special Needs Plans (SNPs) to provide integrated care specifically for individuals who are:

1. institutionalized;
2. Medicare-Medicaid enrollees (dually eligible); and/or
3. experience severe or disabling chronic conditions (SSA, 2003).

Dual Eligible Special Needs Plans (D-SNPs), which serve Medicare and Medicaid enrollees by better coordination of Medicare and Medicaid benefits, provide person-centered care via the identification of barriers to health, understanding each member's needs and preferences, and developing care plans that include community supports. Like other Medicare Advantage plans, SNPs can offer supplemental benefits. The model incorporates a comprehensive health risk assessment to identify the medical, functional, cognitive, psychosocial, and mental health needs of each SNP beneficiary, and the findings are directly incorporated into the development of an individualized care plan and ongoing coordination among the care team and enrollee.

D-SNPs are working creatively to address alignment in providing targeted services and supports to their enrollees in recognition of the fact that strong connectivity with community organizations (e.g., food banks, community health centers, county social services, supportive housing providers, and employment services) is critical to providing whole person care (ACAP, 2020). In one example, a plan is providing a monthly per member payment to a community housing organization that funds housing support services for individuals who meet unstable housing criteria. Early findings show emerging improvements in housing and health outcomes, as well as a decrease in health care spending and utilization once an individual experiences 10 months of stable housing (ACAP, 2020).

D-SNPs are also using technology to better understand enrollees' needs and connect them to whole person care (ACAP, 2020). For example, one D-SNP plan has a team that analyzes data from multiple sources, including population health data, as well as the social and financial impacts of SDoH investments. Another is connecting data across county health services departments to better understand member needs and identify optimal partnership strategies (ACAP, 2020).

The operational coherence among D-SNPs supports greater integration among plans and nonclinical community organizations to provide a full range of care, services, and supports to members. The personalized, data-driven, and coordinated nature of D-SNPs could also influence how health systems approach treatment for people who are not Medicare and Medicaid beneficiaries.

Depending on contexts, states could consider other forms of special needs plans that could provide better care integration for dual eligible beneficiaries. Fully Integrated Dual Eligible Special Needs Plans (FIDE-SNPs) integrate care for beneficiaries under a single managed care organization and cover primary, acute, and long-term services and supports benefits. FIDE-SNPs also cover behavioral health services in most contexts. Meanwhile, Highly Integrated Dual Eligible Special Needs Plans (HIDE-SNPs) include coverage of long-term services and supports benefits, behavioral health services, or both (MACPAC, 2021).

MEDICAID LONG-TERM SERVICES AND SUPPORTS

As the largest payer for long-term care in the country, Medicaid provides coverage of long-term services and supports (LTSS) through a continuum of settings and applies the following principles to promote health (CMS, n.d.-b):

- **Person-driven:** Older people, people with disabilities, and people experiencing chronic illness have the opportunity to decide where and with whom to live, exert control over the services they receive and who provides the services, how to work and earn money, and include friends and supports to help them participate in community life.
- **Inclusive:** The system encourages and supports people to live where they want to live with access to a full array of high-quality, community-based services and supports.
- **Effective and accountable:** High-quality services improve quality of life. Accountability and responsibility are shared among the programs, providers, individuals, and caregivers.
- **Sustainable and efficient:** Economy and efficiency are achieved through the coordination of a personalized package of services in accordance with the individual's needs and goals.

- **Coordinated and transparent:** Services from various funding streams are coordinated to provide a seamless package of supports and make effective use of available technology.
- **Culturally competent:** Services account for cultural and linguistic needs.

Across this long-term care continuum, Medicaid covers a variety of whole person care initiatives through a highly variable collection of home- and community-based services (HCBS) in all 56 states and territories. Medicaid HCBS benefits create the conditions by which older adults and individuals with disabilities can leverage their independence and freedom of choice to receive care in their homes and communities rather than in institutionalized settings such as nursing homes.

Given this choice, individuals have overwhelmingly preferred the option of staying in their own homes and communities. In Medicaid, the majority of long-term care services are now HCBS. As of 2018, 56 percent of Medicaid long-term care consisted of HCBS on the national level, with a few states exceeding 75 percent (CMS, 2021). The $21 billion of investments in HCBS infrastructure in section 9817 of the American Rescue Plan Act will support the payment and delivery of high-quality, cost-effective, whole person care, allowing millions to stay in their homes and communities while receiving high-quality health and social care services and supports (HHS, 2021). Whether this infusion of funds will address concerns that Medicaid LTSS funding does not sufficiently cover the cost of delivering nursing home-level care at home is yet to be determined.

The keystone of HCBS programs is the person-centered plan that addresses health and long-term services and support needs, reflecting the individual's preferences and goals. The person-centered planning process must be directed by the individual, including representatives whom the individual has freely chosen to contribute, and results in a person-centered plan with individually identified goals and preferences that help guide the individual in achieving personally defined outcomes in the most integrated community setting. The plan also ensures the delivery of services in a manner that reflects personal preferences and choices while contributing to the assurance of health and welfare. Some states, like Colorado, provide complementary and integrative health services as part of HCBS, including acupuncture, chiropractic, and massage therapy, including within their spinal cord injury HCBS waiver program. All benefits and services are provided in accordance with the individual's care plan.

Medicaid is by far the largest driver of HCBS services and the largest funder of such care in the country, incurring approximately 57 percent of all HCBS expenditures—an estimated $114 billion in federal FY 2021 (Musumeci, 2021). Other payers have been slow to embrace HCBS, with private insurance covering only 12 percent of the nation's HCBS costs, despite a proven, well-developed, and comprehensive blueprint for providing and monitoring the quality of HCBS in a healthy, safe, and person-centered way (CMS, n.d.-b). A major disincentive is that HCBS rates are often too low, leading to inefficiencies such as the unpayment and overwork of direct-care workers, who are often more likely to belong to a marginalized community (Sullivan, 2021). Moreover, existing HCBS systems are overwhelmed, with hundreds of thousands of people on waiting lists for HCBS across the nation (Sullivan, 2021)—yet another manifestation of our current health crisis. The federal government and private insurance stakeholders must find ways to increase the capacity of HCBS systems, including through sustaining long-term training, career growth, and competitive payment of its providers (Sullivan, 2021).

Aligning policies, programs, and regulations to prioritize the health of individuals and communities remains an uphill task due in significant part to the political realities of federal health care reform today (King, 2017). Despite these challenges, federal legislators, policy practitioners, and health systems can take more incremental actions that circumvent the unfortunate status quo. First, government agencies must be empowered with the statutory authority required to finance, implement, and integrate care models across government departments, such as Medicare and Medicaid. Second, health programs must promote the dignity of people with disabilities through care that leverages independence, freedom of choice, and individual control over their care in both home- and community-based settings. Finally, patients must be better served through meaningful engagement of individuals, health systems, and community-based organizations. These partnerships should collect and apply data to better understand community-specific care needs and preferences, barriers to health, and gaps in services and supports relative to individual and community goals.

Key Pillar 6—Individuals and communities are empowered as organization and delivery decision-makers for matters pertaining to their health.

Engaging and empowering individuals and communities as decision-makers in their own health and the health of their communities is essential to investing in whole person and whole population health. The Community Aging in Place: Advancing Better Living for Elders Model (CAPABLE), Self-Directed Medicaid Services, Collaborative Approach to Public Good Investments, and Federally

Qualified Health Centers are each important examples that adhere to this pillar and provide helpful guidance on the ways in which individual and community empowerment might be centered in efforts for health system transformation.

COMMUNITY AGING IN PLACE: ADVANCING BETTER LIVING FOR ELDERS

Community Aging in Place: Advancing Better Living for Elders (CAPABLE) is a multidisciplinary intervention developed and tested to reduce health disparities among older adults by helping them "age in community." Developed at the Johns Hopkins School of Nursing, CAPABLE teams include an occupational therapist, a nurse, and a handy worker to address the participating older adults' home environment and use their unique strengths to improve independence and safety in their home setting. This program uncovers and leverages intrinsic motivation surrounding what matters to each individual, such as bathing without difficulty, preparing food, or leaving the house and getting into a car for a family event.

Throughout a 4-month service period, CAPABLE members will identify their priorities and goals. Occupational therapists and nurses use a standardized approach tailored to each individual to assess and brainstorm a plan that addresses needs in the individual's home environment. In developing this plan, the team sees the person in their home context, helping to offset biases that might come into play in more traditional clinical settings. Using this plan, a handy worker implements fixes and adaptations (e.g., lighting on the stairs or adaptive cutting boards) according to individual preferences, needs, and clinical expertise.

CAPABLE program sites provide services to older adults without cost, reducing spending on hospital admissions, skilled nursing facility admissions, and specialty care (Szanton, n.d.). Comparing the health care cost expended for participants in CAPABLE to the health care cost for a nonparticipating group, CAPABLE saved, on average, $2,765 per quarter—or more than $10,000 per year—for Medicare for at least 2 years. Inclusive of all patient visits, home repairs, and modifications, CAPABLE costs $2,825 per year while decreasing inpatient and outpatient costs, readmission rates, and observation status stays (Szanton, n.d.).

Despite these successes, CAPABLE is limited in its reach. Only approximately 4,000 older adults have participated in CAPABLE, and an estimated 16.1 million could still benefit from this service when assuming around 35 percent of the 46 million older people above the age of 65 can benefit from home-based interventions due to difficulties with activities of daily living (ACL, 2021; JHU School of Nursing, 2022). To enable access to more supports and services for older people, Medicare could scale and pay for CAPABLE as a Medicare bundle of services, incorporate CAPABLE specifically into value-based care models, or include quality star metrics more clearly to beneficiaries' functional goals.

CAPABLE is currently implemented in 43 sites in 23 states (including rural, frontier, urban, and micropolitan areas) within a variety of policy settings from two accountable care organizations, one hospital readmission project, and a state Medicaid HCBS waiver, as well as in some free-standing clinics and home-based primary care. With American Rescue Plan Act funding, three new states will implement CAPABLE. While the American Rescue Plan Act will enable some scaling of the CAPABLE model, the provided funding and resources will not be sufficient to support the needs of older adults. Through scaling promising models such as CAPABLE, older adults can access care that builds, maintains, and supports physical capacity and independence. Finally, because health remains an essential component to people across all ages, caring for older adults will be integral to a system of whole person, whole population health.

SELF-DIRECTED MEDICAID SERVICES

Self-direction is an expanding and fully person-driven system of care. As of January 2021, 267 programs across the United States empowered more than 1.2 million individuals to direct care resources and services to meet their own needs and preferences (Edwards-Orr et al., 2020). Medicaid is the largest payer of this model, accounting for 66 percent of self-direction funding in 2019, and the VHA is another significant supporter (Edwards-Orr et al., 2020). In 2019, the Veteran-Directed Home and Community Based Services program served more than 2,000 veterans in 71 programs in 41 states.

In self-directed care, participating individuals or their designated caregivers have decision-making authority and take responsibility for managing their services with the assistance of a system of supports. The self-directed service delivery model is an alternative to the traditional service model, such as an agency or health plan responsible for paying for services. Self-direction allows participants to have independence in managing all aspects of service delivery in a person-centered planning process.

Self-direction promotes personal choice and control over the delivery of services, including a choice of who provides the services and how the services are provided. Self-directed care is based on a service plan developed by an individual (with assistance) that identifies individuals' strengths, capacities, preferences, needs, and desired measurable outcomes. While specific services within self-direction vary by state and by program, services are targeted to address problems identified in the individual's service plan, and could include acupuncture, therapeutic horseback riding and equine-assisted activities, hypnotherapy, peer mentoring, art and recreation programs, chiropractic care, massage therapy, family support services, biofeedback, and Native American healers.

In practice, state Medicaid programs provide or arrange for the provision of a system of supports that are responsive to an individual's preferences in developing these plans, managing services and support workers, and performing the responsibilities of an employer. Participants have the authority to recruit, hire, train, and supervise the individuals who provide their services and decide how the Medicaid funds in their budget are spent.

Medicaid has a strong tradition of self-directed care, including Wisconsin's IRIS (Include, Respect, I Self-Direct) program. Since 2008, IRIS has provided self-direction for Medicaid-enrolled frail older adults and adults with disabilities, giving them the freedom to decide how they want to live and allowing for up to 32 services to be self-directed while giving participants full employer and budget authority (WI DHS, 2021). IRIS is built on the belief that everyone holds the potential for meaningful societal contribution, deserves a quality life experience, and has a right to full citizenship (Genz and Urban, 2020). Participants highlight the program's benefits in enhancing independence for individuals and caregiver support to create fuller, healthier, and more meaningful lives. The program has more than 21,000 participants, and its popularity is reinforced by the fact that no waiting list space is available in any of the 72 counties in the state.

COLLABORATIVE APPROACH TO PUBLIC GOOD INVESTMENTS

The Collaborative Approach to Public Good Investments (CAPGI) is a financial model and governance process designed to help multi-stakeholder coalitions sustain new investments in SDoH. This process occurs within communities and uses local capital, stakeholder self-interest, and a collaborative bidding process to source and pay for new services that (1) any single stakeholder could not support and (2) could benefit multiple organizations and the community.

CAPGI is unique because funding for new investments does not rely on third-party private investment capital, which expects to be repaid, or new government expenditures. Rather, it leverages the combined self-interest of existing community partners, some of which may be private or public insurance plans or hospital systems with deep connections to a larger organization. Investing stakeholders could also be local philanthropies, local government, such as law enforcement, and employer or social service organizations. A key feature of the model is the trusted broker, or an organization capable of convening relevant stakeholders, maintaining trust in the confidentiality of their financial bids, and executing the performance contract with the social service provider(s). The deeply interconnected structure of the program, along with the convening power of the trusted broker, is essential to CAPGI's goal of forming partnerships to attract financing for public goods. Additionally, the financing must be sustained over long periods due to the slow yielding nature of CAPGI investments, including increasing access to housing, nutrition, and transportation (Nichols and Taylor, 2018).

Based on a previously developed and modified economic auction model, the novel funding approach was first described in 2018 (Nichols and Taylor, 2018). Currently, three communities are in the first year of using CAPGI—Cleveland, Ohio; Albany, New York; and Waco, Texas—and others are working toward implementation in the next year. The program has attracted commitment and energized involvement from a multi-stakeholder network of cities, states, and communities across racial and ethnic backgrounds, as well as community size. These promising signals indicate that the model has a high likelihood of being scaled to new communities and sustained in existing communities (Nichols et al., 2020). The model is not intended to fix system-wide deficits but could influence future collective action efforts to encourage public good investments that finance social drivers of health infrastructure, including transportation, nutrition, and housing (Nichols and Taylor, 2018).

FEDERALLY QUALIFIED HEALTH CENTERS

Established in 1965 by the federal Office of Economic Opportunity, Federally Qualified Health Centers (FQHCs) aim to deliver integrated, "comprehensive, culturally competent, high-quality primary health care services" (HRSA, 2021b). In exchange for federal grants and special reimbursement by Medicaid and Medicare, FQHCs provide basic health services to all in their geographic community regardless of their ability to pay. In addition to reimbursement for Medicare and Medicaid beneficiaries, FQHCs receive access to 340B discounts on outpatient pharmaceutical products, free vaccines for uninsured and underinsured children, and assistance in recruiting and retaining primary care providers through the National Health Service Corps (HRSA, 2021b).

In exchange for these benefits, and as codified in section 330 of the Public Health Services Act, FQHC entities agree to be organized as nonprofit corporations with their Boards of Directors being:

> composed of individuals, a majority of whom are being served by the center and who, as a group, represent the individuals being served by the center, and

meets at least once a month, selects the services to be provided by the center, schedules the hours during which such services will be provided, approves the center's annual budget, approves the selection of a director for the center, and ... establishes general policies for the center. (United States Code, 2022)

The rationale for insisting on consumer governance in FQHCs is consistent with the sixth pillar for whole person health: to make the organization responsible to the community it serves. By adhering to a community-based, patient-led governance structure, FQHCs also integrate access to pharmacy, mental health, substance use disorders, and oral health services in underserved areas. Access is also improved through health education, translation, transportation, and access to a sliding fee scale (HRSA, 2021b).

Furthermore, FQHCs are able to develop systems of patient-centered and integrated care that can be personalized to diverse populations. These practices include incorporating acupuncture, meditation, tai chi, reiki, mindfulness, and yoga into health programs (Bharath, 2019). A program in Oregon included partnerships to combat food insecurity and health inequities through funding from Medicaid Coordinated Care Organizations, screening through FQHCs, and the distribution of produce from local farmers markets (Kaye, 2021). Some FQHCs, such as the NATIVE project in Spokane, Washington, practice integrating spiritual, cultural, and traditional Native values as part of care. Underpinned by these values, the NATIVE project also prioritizes physical, mental, and emotional health centered alongside education and awareness, drug- and alcohol-free lifestyles, and the integration of mind, body, spirit, and healing paths for patients (NATIVE Project, 2021).

FQHCs now serve more than 30 million people nationwide across the life course, including children, pregnant women, and older adults (HRSA, 2021a). Their patients are disproportionately poor and uninsured, including one in three people living in poverty and one in five rural residents (HRSA, 2021a). With standards of care and service developed, promoted, and enforced by the Health Resources and Services Administration of the Department of Health and Human Services, FQHCs perform as well as or better than privately organized practices serving patients with less complex health care needs (Goldman et al., 2012).

Although the composition of FQHC boards sets this intervention apart from others, its positive performance may not be directly linked to this innovative approach. Moreover, implementing a mechanism that embodies true patient engagement remains a challenge for FQHCs. For example, there remain distinctions between the formal representation of consumers on boards and descriptive representation. There is also the challenge of developing effective governance skills, whether selected consumers are truly representative of community positions, and the power of technical knowledge in board agenda setting (Wright, 2015).

These cautions notwithstanding, with its focus on community governance, public-private partnerships, and active patient participation, consumer-majority health care organization boards as modeled by FQHCs represent a "new governance paradigm" (Campbell, 2011) that challenges traditional models of the governance of large and consolidating nonprofit health systems and exemplifies the sixth pillar of whole person health: communities being empowered as decision-makers in terms of investments intended to benefit their health.

CONCLUSION

While the highlighted models and programs demonstrate the potential of person-centricity, cross-sector collaboration, equity, and aligned financing in achieving better health and well-being, they do not fully achieve the Steering Group's vision of whole person, whole population health. They are vehicles of change and are directionally correct but are not comprehensive, large, or exhaustive enough to effect the change the Steering Group described in Chapters 1 and 2 of this publication.

Although ongoing innovation and work in this space can lead to positive outcomes on smaller scales, the current health and health care system is highly constrained, delaying the transformation required to achieve the Steering Group's vision. Instead, the ideas, innovation, and advances in these models need to be further nurtured and unlocked through leveraging new sources of funding, involving a new and different mix of stakeholders, and scaling the innovative approaches of the presented cases into comprehensive, system-wide change. In the next two chapters, the authors will further discuss the gap between where we are and where we need to be, and highlight the systems-wide action, collaboration, and financing required to achieve the Steering Group's vision of whole person and whole population health.

REFERENCES

ACAP (Association for Community Affiliated Plans). 2020. *Addressing Social Determinants of Health Through Dual-Eligible Special Needs Plans*. Available at: https://www.communityplans.net/research/11927 (accessed April 13, 2022).

ACL (Administration for Community Living). 2021. *2020 Profile of Older Americans*. Available at: https://acl.gov/sites/default/files/aging%20and%20Disability%20In%20America/2020Profileolderamericans.final_.pdf (accessed October 13, 2022).

Bharath, D. 2019. *Integrative Medicine Becomes a Focus for Treating the Uninsured.* Available at: https://centerforhealthjournalism.org/integrative-medicine-becomes-focus-treating-uninsured (accessed August 16, 2022).

Binet, A., G. Rio, M. Arcaya, G. Roderigues, and V. Gavin. 2021. "It feels like money's just flying out the window": Financial security, stress and health in gentrifying neighborhoods. *Cities & Health* 6(3):536-551. https//doi.org/10.1080/23748834.2021.1885250.

Blue Zones. 2022a. *Blue Zones Results Albert Lea, MN.* Available at: https://www.bluezones.com/blue-zones-results-albert-lea-mn/#section-1 (accessed June 21, 2022).

Blue Zones. 2022b. *Blue Zones Project News: Fort Worth's Transformation from One of Unhealthiest Cities in America.* Available at: https://www.bluezones.com/2019/05/blue-zones-project-news-fort-worths-transformation-from-one-of-unhealthiest-cities-in-america (accessed June 21, 2022).

Blumenthal, D., L. Gustaffson, and S. Bishop. 2018. *To Control Health Care Costs, U.S. Employers Should Form Purchasing Alliances.* Available at: https://hbr.org/2018/11/to-control-health-care-costs-u-s-employers-should-form-purchasing-alliances (accessed October 12, 2022).

Bokhour, B. G., J. N. Haun, J. Hyde, M. Charns, and B. Kligler. 2020a. Transforming the Veterans Affairs to a whole health system of care: Time for action and research. *Medical Care* 58(4):295-300. https//doi.org/10.1097/MLR.0000000000001316.

Bokhour B. G., J. K. Hyde, S. Zeliadt, and D. C. Mohr. 2020b. *Whole Health System of Care Evaluation—A Progress Report on Outcomes of the WHS Pilot at 18 Flagship Sites. Veterans Health Administration, Center for Evaluating Patient-Centered Care in VA (EPCC-VA).* Available at: https://www.va.gov/WHOLEHEALTH/professional-resources/clinician-tools/Evidence-Based-Research.asp (accessed October 12, 2022).

Build Healthy Places Network. 2021. *Intermountain Healthcare & the Utah Housing Preservation Fund.* Available at: https://buildhealthyplaces.org/sharing-knowledge/publications/community-close-ups/intermountain-healthcare-the-utah-housing-preservation-fund (accessed October 13, 2022).

Business Insider. 2018. *Southcentral Foundation Accepts Second Malcolm Baldrige Award.* Available at: https://markets.businessinsider.com/news/stocks/southcentral-foundation-accepts-second-malcolm-baldrige-award-1021346598 (accessed June 21, 2022).

Campbell, Y. 2011. New governance in action: Community health centers and the Public Health Service Act. *St. Louis University Journal of Health Law and Policy*

4(2). Available at: https://scholarship.law.slu.edu/jhlp/vol4/iss2/6 (accessed June 21, 2022).

Church, M. S. 2018. *Investing in Health from the Ground Up: Building a Market for Healthy Neighborhoods*. Available at: https://investinresults.org/sites/default/files/book-chapter/WM_29_Super-Church_0.pdf (accessed August 11, 2022).

Church, M. S., and J. Flatley. 2020. *Healthy Neighborhoods Equity Fund II: Theory of Change*. Available at: https://static1.squarespace.com/static/5f31ae81bcb71e20e39311bb/t/5f875712a87a740f5b668f48/1602705172416/HNEF+II+ToC+Full+Text+Final+06.02.20.pdf (accessed August 11, 2022).

Church, M. S., and K. McGilvray. 2018. Improving health and environment through place-based investing: The Healthy Neighborhoods Equity Fund. *Journal of Affordable Housing & Community Development Law* 27(2):353-366. https://www.jstor.org/stable/26496809.

CMS (Centers for Medicare & Medicaid Services). 2011. *Chapter 13 Payments to PACE Organizations*. Available at: https://www.cms.gov/Regulations-and-Guidance/Guidance/Manuals/Downloads/pace111c13.pdf (accessed April 6, 2022).

CMS. 2021. *Medicaid Long Term Services and Supports Annual Expenditures Report: Federal Fiscal Years 2017 and 2018*. Available at: https://www.medicaid.gov/medicaid/long-term-services-supports/downloads/ltssexpenditures-2017-2018.pdf (accessed April 6, 2022).

CMS. n.d.-a. *Programs of All-Inclusive Care for the Elderly Benefits*. Available at: https://www.medicaid.gov/medicaid/long-term-services-supports/pace/programs-all-inclusive-care-elderly-benefits/index.html (accessed April 6, 2022).

CMS. n.d.-b. *Long Term Services and Supports*. Available at: https://www.medicaid.gov/medicaid/long-term-services-supports/index.html (accessed April 6, 2022).

CMS. n.d.-c. *Independence at Home Demonstration*. Available at: https://innovation.cms.gov/innovation-models/independence-at-home (accessed June 21, 2022).

Community Preventive Services Task Force. 2015. *School-Based Health Centers*. Available at: https://www.thecommunityguide.org/sites/default/files/assets/OnePager-SBHC.pdf (accessed June 21, 2022).

Conservation Law Foundation. 2021. *HealthScore Metrics That Matter for Healthy and Resilient Neighborhoods*. Available at: https://www.clf.org/wp-content/uploads/2021/12/CLF-HealthScore-WEB.pdf (accessed July 28, 2022).

County Health Rankings & Roadmaps. 2023. *2023 County Health Rankings National Findings Report*. Available at: https://www.countyhealthrankings.org/reports/2023-county-health-rankings-national-findings-report (accessed May 15, 2023).

Dana-Farber Cancer Institute. 2021. *Healthy Neighborhoods Fund Gets Major Boost.* Available at: https://www.dana-farber.org/newsroom/news-releases/2021/healthy-neighborhoods-fund-gets-major-boost (accessed August 11, 2022).

Edwards-Orr, M., M. Morris, C. DeLuca, K. Ujvari, and M. Sciegaj. 2020. *National Inventory of Self-Directed Long-Term Services and Supports Programs.* Available at: https://www.longtermscorecard.org/publications/promising-practices/2019-self-directed-ltss-inventory (accessed June 21, 2022).

Genz, B., and S. Urban. 2020. *IRIS Self-Directed Personal Care: Gateway to Community and a Self-Determined Life.* Available at: http://www.advancingstates.org/sites/nasuad/files/u24453/Self-Directed%20Personal%20Care%20Gateway%20to%20Community%20and%20a%20Self-Determined%20Life.pdf (accessed April 11, 2022).

Goetzel, R. Z., E. C. Roemer, C. Holingue, M. D. Fallin, K. McCleary, W. Eaton, J. Agnew, F. Azocar, D. Ballard, J. Bartlett, M. Braga, H. Conway, K. A. Crighton, R. Frank, K. Jinnett, D. Kellar-Greene, S. M. Rauch, R. Safeer, D. Saporito, A. Schill, D. Shern, V. Strecher, P. Wald, P. Wang, and C. R. Mattingly. 2018. Mental health in the workplace: A call to action proceedings from the mental health in the workplace: Public health summit. *Journal of Occupational and Environmental Medicine* 60(4):322-330.

Goetzel, R. Z., R. M. Henke, M. A. Head, R. Benevent, and K. Rhee. 2020. Ten modifiable health risk factors and employees' medical costs—An update. *American Journal of Health Promotion* 34(5):490-499.

Goldman, L. E., P. W. Chu, H. Tran, M. J. Romano, and R. S. Stafford. 2012. Federally Qualified Health Centers and private practice performance on ambulatory care measures. *American Journal of Preventive Medicine* 43(2):142-149. https://doi.org/10.1016/j.amepre.2012.02.033.

Gottlieb, K. 2013. The Nuka System of Care: Improving health through ownership and relationships. *International Journal of Circumpolar Health* 72. https://doi.org/10.3402/ijch.v72i0.21118.

Gottlieb, K., I. Sylvester, and D. Eby. 2008. Transforming your practice: What matters most. *Family Practice Management* 15(1):32.

Harvard Project. 2015. *School-Based Health Centers: Fort Peck Assiniboine and Sioux Tribes.* Available at: https://hwpi.harvard.edu/files/hpaied/files/schoolbasedhealthcenters-final_2.pdf?m=1639579174 (accessed July 15, 2022).

Healthcare Anchor Network. 2022. *Healthcare Anchor Network.* Available at: https://healthcareanchor.network (accessed October 13, 2022).

HHS (U.S. Department of Health and Human Services). 2021. *CMS Issues Guidance on American Rescue Plan Funding for Medicaid Home and Community Based Services.* Available at: https://www.hhs.gov/about/news/2021/05/13/

cms-issues-guidance-american-rescue-plan-funding-medicaid-home-and-community-based-services.html (accessed April 6, 2022).
HNEF (Healthy Neighborhood Equity Fund). 2020. *Transformative Impacts of Healthy Neighborhoods Equity Fund I*. Available at: https://static1.squarespace.com/static/5f31ae81bcb71e20e39311bb/t/5f641b3640e1a14ef6b3c9e5/1600396097669/HNEF+Impact+Infographic+Final+02.14.20.pdf (accessed August 11, 2022).
HNEF. 2022a. *Investment*. Available at: https://www.hnefund.org/investment (accessed July 28, 2022).
HNEF. 2022b. *Eligibility & Screening*. Available at: https://www.hnefund.org/eligibilityscreening (accessed July 28, 2022).
HRSA (Health Resources and Services Administration). 2021a. *Health Center Program: Impact and Growth*. Available at: https://bphc.hrsa.gov/about-health-centers/health-center-program-impact-growth (accessed August 16, 2022).
HRSA. 2021b. *What Is a Health Center?* Available at: https://bphc.hrsa.gov/about-health-centers/what-health-center (accessed August 16, 2022).
IOM (Institute of Medicine). 2015. *Business Engagement in Building Healthy Communities: Workshop Summary*. Washington, DC: The National Academies Press.
Jain, A., J. Levy, D. Polsky, and K. E. Anderson. 2022. Medicare Advantage and the Maryland all-payer model. *Health Affairs Forefront* March 18. https://doi.org/10.1377/forefront.20220316.50044.
JHU (Johns Hopkins University) School of Nursing. 2022. *CAPABLE FAQs*. Available at: https://nursing.jhu.edu/faculty_research/research/projects/capable/capable-faqs.html (accessed October 12, 2022).
Kaye, N. 2021. *Oregon's Community Care Organization 2.0 Fosters Community Partnerships to Address Social Determinants of Health*. Available at: https://www.nashp.org/oregons-community-care-organization-2-0-fosters-community-partnerships-to-address-social-determinants-of-health/#toggle-id-6 (accessed August 16, 2022).
King, M. W. 2017. Health Care Efficiencies: Consolidation and Alternative Models vs. Health Care and Antitrust Regulation—Irreconcilable Differences? *American Journal of Law & Medicine* 43(4):426-467. https://doi.org/10.1177/0098858817753407.
Larson, S. 2021. *What's Different When the Community Collects the Data?* Available at: https://shelterforce.org/2021/08/10/what-happens-when-the-community-collects-the-data (accessed August 11, 2022).
Machta, R., G. Peterson, J. Rotter, K. Stewart, S. Heitkamp, I. Platt, D. Whicher, K. Calkins, K. Krankler, L. Barterian, and N. McCall. *Evaluation of the Maryland*

Total Cost of Care Model: Implementation Report. Available at: https://www.mathematica.org/publications/evaluation-of-the-maryland-total-cost-of-care-model-implementation-report (accessed June 21, 2022).

MACPAC. 2018. *Medicaid in Schools*. Available at: https://www.macpac.gov/wp-content/uploads/2018/04/Medicaid-in-Schools.pdf (accessed June 21, 2022).

MACPAC. 2021. *Medicare Advantage Dual Eligible Special Needs Plans*. Available at: https://www.macpac.gov/subtopic/medicare-advantage-dual-eligible-special-needs-plans-aligned-with-medicaid-managed-long-term-services-and-supports (accessed March 16, 2023).

Mattke, S., K. Kapinos, J. P. Caloyeras, E. A. Taylor, B. Batorsky, H. Liu, K. R. Van Busum, and S. Newberry. 2015. Workplace wellness programs: Services offered, participation, and incentives. *RAND Health Quarterly* 5(2).

Medicaid. n.d. *Program of All-Inclusive Care for the Elderly*. Available at: https://www.medicaid.gov/medicaid/long-term-services-supports/program-all-inclusive-care-elderly/index.html (accessed October 12, 2022).

Murray, R. 2009. Setting hospital rates to control costs and boost quality: The Maryland experience. *Health Affairs* 28(5):1395-1405.

Musumeci, M. 2021. *How Could $400 Billion New Federal Dollars Change Medicaid Home and Community-Based Services?* Available at: https://www.kff.org/medicaid/issue-brief/how-could-400-billion-new-federal-dollars-change-medicaid-home-and-community-based-services (accessed August 16, 2022).

NATIVE Project. 2021. *About Us*. Available at: https://nativeproject.org/about-us (accessed August 16, 2022).

Nichols, L. M., and L. A. Taylor. 2018. Social determinants as public goods: A new approach to financing key investments in healthy communities. *Health Affairs* 37(8):1223-1230.

Nichols, L., L. Taylor, P. Hughes-Cromwick, G. Miller, A. Turner, C. Rhyan, and R. Hamrick. 2020. Collaborative Approach To Public Goods Investments (CAPGI): Lessons learned from a feasibility study. *Health Affairs Blog*, August 13. https://doi.org/10.1377/forefront.20200811.667525.

NIST (National Institute of Standards and Technology). 2017. *Southcentral Foundation: Malcolm Baldrige National Quality Award 2011 Award Recipient Health Care*. Available at: https://www.nist.gov/baldrige/southcentral-foundation (accessed June 21, 2022).

NRC (National Research Center). 2019. *Complementary and Integrative Health Services Evaluation: Annual Report SFY 2018-19*. Available at: https://hcpf.colorado.gov/sites/hcpf/files/NRC%20Annual%20Report%20to%20HCPF%20SFY1819-June%202019.pdf (accessed April 6, 2022).

NYC DOE (New York City Department of Education). 2022. *School-Based Health Centers*. Available at: https://www.schools.nyc.gov/school-life/health-and-wellness/school-based-health-centers (accessed June 21, 2022).

PACE (National PACE Association). 2020. *PACE by the Numbers*. Available at: https://www.npaonline.org/sites/default/files/images/NPA%20infographic%203%20%2020%20%281%29.pdf (accessed April 6, 2022).

PACE. 2022. *The History of PACE*. Available at: https://www.npaonline.org/policy-advocacy/value-pace (accessed April 5, 2022).

Quantified Ventures. 2021a. *Drug Free Moms and Babies Program*. Available at: https://www.quantifiedventures.com/drug-free-moms-and-babies-program (accessed August 18, 2022).

Quantified Ventures. 2021b. *Hope Has a Home Medical Respite Program*. Available at: https://www.quantifiedventures.com/hope-has-a-home-medical-respite-program (accessed August 18, 2022).

Quantified Ventures. 2021c. *Together in Care Meal Delivery Program*. Available at: https://www.quantifiedventures.com/together-in-care-meal-delivery-program (accessed August 18, 2022).

Reddy, K. P., T. M. Schult, A. M. Whitehead, and B. G. Bokhour. 2021. Veterans Health Administration's whole health system of care: Supporting the health, well-being, and resiliency of employees. *Global Advances in Health and Medicine* 10:21649561211022698. https://doi.org/10.1177/21649561211022698.

RTI (RTI International). 2019. *Evaluation of the Maryland All-Payer Model*. Available at: https://downloads.cms.gov/files/md-allpayer-finalevalrpt.pdf (accessed May 19, 2022).

Salinsky, E. 2017. *The Nuka System of Care*. Available at: https://scfnuka.com/wp-content/uploads/2016/09/NUKA-CaseStudy.pdf (accessed June 21, 2022).

Sapra, K. J., K. Wunderlich, and H. Haft. 2019. Maryland total cost of care model: Transforming health and health care. *JAMA* 321(10):939-940.

Sholl, J. n.d. *The Profits of a Healthy Workplace*. Available at: https://experiencelife.lifetime.life/article/the-profits-of-a-healthy-workplace (accessed June 2, 2022).

Southcentral Foundation. 2017. *Malcolm Baldrige National Quality Award 2017 Application*. Available at: https://www.baldrigeinstitute.org/HigherLogic/System/DownloadDocumentFile.ashx?DocumentFileKey=cd2dbc11-58b5-97b8-4d8f-6432ff6b5e3f&forceDialog=0 (accessed June 21, 2022).

Southcentral Foundation. n.d. *About Us: NUKA FAQs*. Available at: https://scfnuka.com/about-us/#toggle-id-6 (accessed June 21, 2022).

SSA (Social Security Administration). 2003. *Medicare Modernization Act*. Available at: https://www.ssa.gov/privacy/pia/Medicare%20Modernization%20Act%20(MMA)%20FY07.htm (accessed October 13, 2022).

Sullivan, J. 2021. *States Are Using One-Time Funds to Improve Medicaid Home- and Community-Based Services, But Longer-Term Investments Are Needed*. Available at: https://www.cbpp.org/research/health/states-are-using-one-time-funds-to-improve-medicaid-home-and-community-based (accessed October 13, 2022).

Szanton, S. n.d. *Community Aging in Place: Advancing Better Living for Elders (CAPABLE)*. Available at: https://www.aannet.org/initiatives/edge-runners/profiles/edge-runners--community-aging-place (accessed June 23, 2023).

The King's Fund. n.d. *Nuka System of Care, Alaska*. Available at: https://www.kingsfund.org.uk/publications/population-health-systems/nuka-system-care-alaska (accessed March 22, 2023).

Thomson Reuters. 2011. *Evaluation of Practice Models for Dual Eligibles and Medicare Beneficiaries with Serious Chronic Conditions*. Available at: https://www.cms.gov/Research-Statistics-Data-and-Systems/Statistics-Trends-and-Reports/Medicare-Geographic-Variation/Downloads/PACESiteVisitReport.pdf (accessed April 6, 2022).

United States Code. 2022. *254b. Health Centers*. Available at: https://uscode.house.gov/view.xhtml?req=granuleid:USC-prelim-title42-section254b&num=0&edition=prelim (accessed August 16, 2022).

UnitedHealth Group. 2022. *UnitedHealth Group Commits $25 Million to New England Healthy Neighborhoods Fund*. Available at: https://www.unitedhealthgroup.com/newsroom/2022/2022-07-12-uhg-commits-25mil-to-healthy-neighborhood-fund.html (accessed June 23, 2023).

U.S. Impact Investing Alliance. 2021. *Impact in Place: Emerging Sources of Community Investment Capital and Strategies to Direct it at Scale*. Available at: https://www.newyorkfed.org/medialibrary/media/outreach-and-education/community-development/emerging-sources-of-community-investment/community-investing-bank-report-final-20210518 (accessed August 17, 2022).

VA (U.S. Department of Veterans Affairs). 2021. *Whole Health Circle of Health*. https://www.va.gov/WHOLEHEALTH/circle-of-health/index.asp (accessed March 28, 2022).

VA. 2022. *Whole Health*. https://www.va.gov/wholehealth (accessed March 28, 2022).

Whitehead, A. M., B. Kligler. 2020. Innovations in care: Complementary and integrative health in the Veterans Health Administration whole health system. *Medical Care* 58:S78-S79.

WI DHS (Wisconsin Department of Health Services). 2021. *Include, Respect, I Self-Direct*. Available at: https://www.dhs.wisconsin.gov/iris/index.htm (accessed April 11, 2022).

Wright, B. 2015. Voices of the vulnerable: Community health centers and the promise and peril of consumer governance. *Public Management Review* 17(1):57-71. https://doi.org/10.1080/14719037.2014.881537.

4

INVESTMENT GOALS AND PRIORITY ACTIONS

The examples described in Chapter 3 illustrate that approaches to whole person and population health can be successful when supported by complementary financial strategies and partnerships. The Steering Group largely agreed that global, capitated, and total cost of care payment models is the best platform to facilitate the implementation of comprehensive health and social services that promote population health. However, the right payment infrastructure—cohesive financial reforms and policy alignment—is needed to sustain and scale these models. Ultimately, the nation must pay for the right services at the right price and in the right way.

GOALS

The Steering Group held numerous discussions on the urgent possibilities for the future of health in the United States, from which an emphasis on creating goals arose organically. The Steering Group has summarized the following goals as both important and possible to achieve by 2030 if the will is marshaled by the critical stakeholders. Specifically, the Steering Group feels that by 2030, all U.S. stakeholders, including but not limited to the health system, should be able to build a system reflecting a commitment to whole person, whole population health by:

1. Reducing by 50 percent public and private expenditures that are currently spent on health care services and processes that do not improve health.

The United States should stop paying for services that do not improve health. Previous IOM reports, including *The Healthcare Imperative: Lowering Costs and Improving Outcomes* (IOM, 2010), and subsequent follow-up studies (Berwick and Hackbarth, 2012; Shrank et al., 2019) estimate the cost of waste in the U.S.

health care system (i.e., services that are provided to individuals and paid for but have no impact on their health and well-being) ranges from $760 billion to $935 billion, which accounts for nearly 25 percent of U.S. health care spending (Bauchner and Fontanarosa, 2019). This waste manifests through the delivery of fragmented, low-value, and excessive care, pricing failures, fraud and abuse, and excessive administrative complexity, and must be eliminated from the American health system (Lallemand, 2012).

Successfully addressing these sources of waste could reduce health care spending by more than $200 billion annually, thereby freeing up funding for better, more holistic interventions and providing better and more comprehensive care at lower costs (Shrank et al., 2019). Similar efforts, such as those taken by the One Percent Steps for Healthcare Reform, have identified tangible areas for action, such as capping provider prices and price growth, reducing waste in long-term care hospitals, and reforming home health care coverage to reduce fraud, that could yield an estimated $350 billion annually (One Percent Steps for Health Care Reform, 2022).

2. Increasing by 50 percent public and private expenditures on social interventions that have been proven to improve health.

The United States must improve payment for services and providers that have been shown to advance whole health. This transformation must begin with formal recognition of the value of upstream services and programs that address social determinants of health (SDoH), such as access to stable, quality housing, nutritious food, and vocational support. These services and programs are critical to achieving whole health, and they must extend to the redesign of incentive structures to reward the full spectrum of team-based and multidisciplinary care.

The United States has the lowest ratio of social-to-health care spending among Organisation for Economic Co-operation and Development (OECD) countries. For every $1 spent on health care in the United States, about $0.90 is spent on social services. Meanwhile, in other OECD countries, for every $1 spent on health care, an average of $2 is spent on social services (NASEM, 2019). OECD countries that spend a higher proportion of their gross domestic product (GDP) on social services than on health care—including Germany, Japan, and the United Kingdom—have better health outcomes than those that do not, as described in Chapter 1 (Bradley et al., 2017; Rubin et al., 2016). This fact also holds true within the United States. States with higher ratios of social-to-health spending, including Washington, New Mexico, and Vermont, also appear to have better health outcomes than those with lower ratios (Bradley et al., 2016).

Because the United States experiences serious levels of wealth inequality, poverty, and structural racism, increasing social spending (the lack of which has been a structural driver of poor health in the nation) would enhance health outcomes significantly (Avanceña et al., 2021).

Many of the models described in Chapter 3 have been proven to generate better health outcomes when compared to fee-for-service-dependent care. A substantial driver of this success includes their investment of more resources in social services that can positively influence the upstream SDoH and reduce downstream health care costs. Effective care models should invest in health-promoting interventions and care providers that make the most robust difference in the health and well-being of individuals and populations, including:

- Preventive services across the life span, particularly when implemented early in life, that will produce compounding returns on the health and well-being of the population served (Fried, 2016). For historically marginalized populations, this especially applies to interventions that address social needs and risk factors, starting at a young age and continuing through adulthood (NASEM, 2019).
- A life-course approach that intervenes throughout the national ecosystem—from households and educational institutions to health systems and community-based organizations—that supports whole person, whole population health and well-being. More important are the operational challenges of funding, measuring, and learning such interventions so that they are scaled through whole ecosystems.
- Screening and prevention through the expansion of Medicaid's Early and Periodic Screening, Diagnostic, and Treatment (EPSDT) benefit beyond children under the age of 21 to larger portions of the U.S. population. The EPSDT benefit is representative of whole health through its emphasis on promoting health, proactively screening for disease, and early treatment. Policies across sectors that prevent disease, tackle systemic racism, and assume a life-course approach to disease prevention and health promotion would help stem the crisis of our nation's health.
- Flexible, multimodal approaches to clinical services that are designed to enhance access, improve outcomes, and meet the unique health, social, and long-term care needs of individuals, families, and communities throughout their life spans.
- Community-based organizations and nontraditional service providers (see Box 3), which are often better suited to operationalize and implement whole health interventions than traditional health care providers. These providers should be recognized through funding and integration into whole person and whole population health interventions, including primary care, as

> **BOX 3**
>
> *Innovative Whole Person and Whole Population Health Service Providers*
>
> - Peer counselors and navigators
> - Community health workers and promotores de salud
> - Caregivers, including family members and friends
> - Professionals who offer complementary and integrative therapies (e.g., acupuncture, yoga, meditation)
> - Child life professionals
> - Community-based organization network coordinators
> - Perinatal support specialists (e.g., doulas)
> - Social workers
> - Digital health navigators

recommended by the 2021 National Academies report *Implementing High-Quality Primary Care* (NASEM, 2021a).

3. Utilizing population-based global budgets across all payers to ensure that at least 50 percent of the U.S. population has access to the broad range of social interventions necessary to attain and maintain health and well-being.

A global budget provides a fixed amount of funding to an accountable entity for the totality of services associated with the care of a specified population over a fixed time, rather than payment for individual services or cases. This payment approach provides a foundation that enables the redistribution of current health care spending toward services that have been shown to advance population health and well-being, as outlined in Goals 1 and 2. These prospective population-based payments also offer providers financial resilience in the face of crises like the COVID-19 pandemic, allow for more flexible care delivery models, and allow for the integration of medical and social services (Gondi and Choksi, 2020; Levy et al., 2021).

Global budgets have supported the innovation behind the U.S. Department of Veterans Affairs' (VA's) Whole Health model of care as well as Southcentral Foundation's Nuka System of Care, which are both featured as case studies in Chapter 3. As previously described, the Nuka System of Care offers a full continuum of care (including prevention, behavioral health, primary care, and supportive services) with a substantial portion of the operating revenue flowing from the federal Indian Health Service through a mechanism that functions like a global budget. Funding independent of service volume empowers Nuka's integrated care delivery, allowing for more holistic care associated with positive health outcomes.

Thus, global budgeting should be the primary financing structure used by organizations capable of accepting total accountability for the needs and outcomes that matter to individuals, families, and communities. In scenarios where global budgeting is not applicable, such as due to organizational structure or program type, the ideas behind global budgeting can be approximated using creatively braided and blended financing streams to ensure that adequate, non-siloed funding is in place to support a holistic set of services designed to benefit whole person and population health.

As of 2018, only 5 percent of health care payments to service providers were population-based, although global budgets have also been implemented in a few states, such as Maryland and Vermont (NASEM, 2021b; Shrank et al., 2021). Over the last decade, the Center for Medicare & Medicaid Innovation (CMMI) has launched multiple value-based payment models with mixed results, with global budget demonstrations performing best among them (Smith, 2021). However, most of these models have not been mandatory nor required large shifts away from fee-for-service. As a result, their impact on cost and outcomes has been limited (Crook et al., 2021).

4. Tying 75 percent of health care provider and plan revenues to performance metrics based on the most important health and well-being outcomes, according to the goals of the populations being served.

Accountability measures should align with the health and well-being outcomes that matter most to individuals, families, and communities. To reverse the declining health of our society, it is imperative to think beyond short-term financial returns and process indicators that do not equate to health outcomes valued by individuals, families, and communities, but on which our current quality measurement system overly relies. For instance, clinicians must evolve beyond asking patients, "Do you feel depressed?" to patient-centered questions such as "Have you stopped feeling suicidal? Are you able to take care of yourself (i.e., bathe, get dressed, and eat healthy foods), go to work, be with your family, etc.?" To ensure that financial incentives are aligned with what matters to individuals, families, and communities, quality measures must focus on patient-centered priorities, e.g., validated functional and patient-reported outcome measures (Burstin et al., 2017).

There must be a fundamental alignment between the health system's economic success and the community's health, as defined by the community.

Strategies should also be deployed for the broad engagement of individuals, especially those from historically marginalized populations, in developing a series of measures that increase the overall accountability of health and health care providers to those they serve. These measures should assess and center health equity within the community and specify the key components for high-quality care for diverse and historically marginalized populations, such as health literacy, language access, and cultural competence. As the National Center for Quality Assurance suggests, measures to evaluate a health care organization based on a broader patient-centered framework could also include measures of healthy organizational culture and values, workforce diversity, community engagement activities, and patient engagement efforts (Bau et al., 2019). Furthermore, measurement data should be stratified to identify and track the existence of inequities across factors such as race, ethnicity, geography, disability, and income. An example of this work is CMMI's recent identification of implicit bias in assessing health and risk status, model selection criteria, and the overall demographics of model participants. Mitigating the impact of this bias and more accurately accounting for the needs and outcomes for marginalized populations will be critical to achieving the Steering Group's vision (Majerol and Hughes, 2022).

Rigorous measurement approaches should proactively identify any characteristics of care that systematically exclude individuals or treat populations inequitably. Where algorithms or artificial intelligence is applied, careful consideration in design and evaluation is required to ensure bias across race, income, geographic location, and other factors is minimized to promote equitable resource allocation and access to health care. Properly applied, measurement practices could inform continuous learning models to identify best practices that can be spread and scaled broadly.

To achieve individual health and well-being, incentives cannot stop at the exit door of the health care system. They must extend to the community and social contexts that also shape people's health. At its most comprehensive level, such a system must also reward approaches that improve the health of people who do not engage with the health care system due to lack of access, financial barriers, or deep-seated mistrust rooted in historical trauma. The financing and payment system must support equitable health care that links all people, not just patients, to resources that meet their health-related social needs along with their medical needs, regardless of payer or socio-demographic group. This system should also encourage health care organizations to engage with their respective communities to tackle major threats to health, such as homelessness, poverty, violence, and racism.

5. Substantially enhancing community health engagement and focus as reflected by progress in at least 50 of the 100 counties with the worst health status (as defined by years of potential life lost)—specifically, the success of stakeholders in:
- **Establishing a community-governed, multi-stakeholder coalition that engages those with the greatest health risks in key decisions around allocating community resources;**
- **Achieving a 50 percent improvement in key health and well-being–related indicators deemed important by the coalitions mentioned above; and**
- **Closing the gap on disparities in selected health and well-being indicators across racial/ethnic groups, socioeconomic strata, and disability status.**

Ultimately, if the goal is to improve health, the most needed step is to redirect resources and attention to the communities experiencing the worst outcomes. Individuals in these communities should have a voice in deciding which indicators to use for assessing health and well-being and be empowered to participate in multi-stakeholder deliberations on how to direct resources to improve these indicators. Those with the greatest health risks and historically marginalized communities (e.g., low income, rural, communities of color, and people with disabilities) should not only be represented but also have shared decision-making authority in community governance structures.

Examples of whole person and whole population health measures that community stakeholders could adopt include maternal or infant mortality, suicide rates, employment, educational attainment, self-reported health status, or patient-reported outcomes. Additionally, local cross-sector collaborations with defined accountability, community governance, and aligned incentives will be needed to improve the health and well-being of communities. Such structures are highly effective (as described in the Collaborative Approach to Public Goods Investments model in Chapter 3) and allow for private and public organizations (including federal agencies, such as the Centers for Medicare & Medicaid Services) that might work in siloes to meaningfully partner and coordinate care and services as a united team.

Multi-stakeholder community collaborations could include leaders from community member groups, grassroots community-based organizations, county and municipal government agencies, health care entities, employers, and local community foundations. These stakeholders should be deeply invested in identifying and addressing community needs. They must also provide the lived experiences and perspectives necessary to include and elevate diverse consumer voices in designing solutions. Figure 4 illustrates key components of such collaborations as described throughout this report.

Furthermore, state governments, health care providers, and health plans must partner with these community collaborations and strengthen community infrastructures to achieve health and health equity for all community members. An example of this collaboration can be found in the work of West Side United, a community convener and pooled financing manager in Chicago, Illinois. Community infrastructure can enable communities to be efficient and operate at scale through community governance that facilitates shared goals and outcomes, community governance, workforce development, use of technology, sharing health data, analytics, as well as technical assistance to build and strengthen the capacity of local community-based organizations.

WHOLE PERSON, WHOLE POPULATION HEALTH AND WELL-BEING

LOCAL MULTI-SOURCE BENEFIT FUNDS

COMMUNITY WELL-BEING METRICS

WELL-BEING EXTENSION SERVICE

COMMUNITY WELL-BEING COALITIONS

WELL-BEING METRICS AND INDEX

LOCAL CROSS-SECTOR COMMUNITY GOVERNANCE

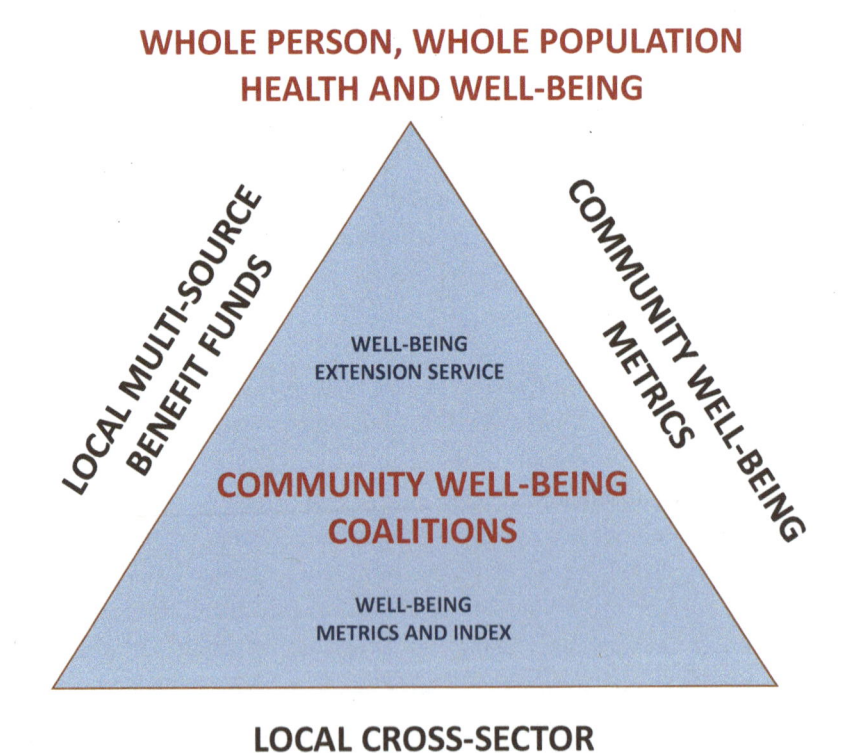

FIGURE 4 | Key components of multi-stakeholder community collaborations.

OPPORTUNITIES FOR STAKEHOLDER ACTION

The following section provides specific actions stakeholders can take to advance whole person and whole population health. Key stakeholders include:

- Patients, families, and communities
- State and local governments
    - Legislative and executive branches
    - Community benefit oversight
    - Insurance oversight
    - Public health agencies and departments
- Federal government
- Care delivery organizations and health systems
- Payers
- Employers
- Financial sector organizations

The Steering Group advocates for transformational change that will lead to meaningful reform in the health investment landscape. While incremental progress is helpful, these actions are unlikely to enable us to meet the above stated goals by 2030 and are, therefore, insufficient. Transformative change is necessary and will move the nation forward on the critical path to better health. In this context, the stakeholder actions are characterized as either transformative or intermediate/incremental.

Patients, Families, and Communities

Patients, families, and communities have a critical role in reversing the nation's declining health trajectory through their lived experiences and power as voters and consumers of care. As demonstrated by the climate change movement, a broad-based grassroots movement will be necessary to push leaders to prioritize health above entrenched interests and to sustain the political will for change. As Daniel Dawes writes, the "political determinants of health," or the relative empowerment across communities to participate in voting, governing, and otherwise influencing policy making, play an outsized role in creating a healthy and inclusive society (Erdelack, 2020).

Transformative Action

- Harness the political process and advocate for financial reforms and more equitable and inclusive health policies.

Intermediate and Incremental Actions

- Engage in advocacy skills training to enhance the power of the whole person, whole population health movement by expanding stakeholder networks. These activities could include educative, community-based public forums that increase civic engagement, improve health literacy, and provide lessons on effectively engaging policy makers and other public officials. New Orleans, Louisiana, and Charlotte, North Carolina, are two examples of cities that provide free training that helps residents build the necessary skills to improve quality of life in their communities.
- Develop and participate in community-based, multi-stakeholder coalitions to guide the design, implementation, and evaluation of programs to support whole person and whole population health and well-being.
- Ensure that a diverse array of community members is involved in the governance of local, state, and/or regional health coalitions to improve equity, inclusion, and representation as it pertains to race, ethnicity, age, and disability status, among other personal characteristics.
- Educate stakeholders on the need to advocate for policies that prioritize whole health, including the indirect impacts of other policy decisions on health.

The following table provides an overview of the Steering Group's judgment of the impact and feasibility of the priority actions described above.

Priority Action	Category	Impact Rating (1 to 5) 1-least impactful; 5-most impactful	Feasibility Rating (1 to 5) 1-least feasible; 5-most feasible
Harness the political process and advocate for financial reforms and more equitable and inclusive health policies.	Transformative	4.4	2.6
Engage in advocacy skills training to enhance the power of the whole person, whole population health movement by expanding stakeholder networks.	Intermediate and Incremental	2.8	3.6

Develop and participate in community-based, multi-stakeholder coalitions to guide the design, implementation, and evaluation of programs to support whole person and whole population health and well-being.	Intermediate and Incremental	3.2	3.4
Ensure that a diverse array of community members is involved in the governance of local, state, and/or regional health coalitions to improve equity, inclusion, and representation as it pertains to race, ethnicity, age, and disability status, among other personal characteristics.	Intermediate and Incremental	3	3.2
Educate stakeholders on the need to advocate for policies that prioritize whole health, including the indirect impacts of other policy decisions on health.	Intermediate and Incremental	2.8	3.6

State and Local Governments

Legislative and Executive Branches. State governments finance significant portions of health care through their Medicaid and public employee benefit programs that are directed and regulated by General Assemblies and relevant agencies. Decisions under the purview of these legislative and executive governing bodies, such as which services they pay for and how they negotiate contracts with health plans and providers, can significantly impact the health and well-being of state residents, making them important influencers of whole person and population health.

Transformative Actions

- Pursue and use 1115 waivers to cover innovative care and payment models that address social determinants of health. This waiver enables services determined by the state to be medically appropriate and cost-effective substitutes for covered services or settings under state Medicaid plans (OHA, 2023). Recent innovations in applying 1115 waivers include health-related social needs such as food-as-medicine interventions, safe housing, and water pollution (Held, 2022).
- Require managed care organizations to focus on prevention and social determinants of health through Medicaid managed care contracts. Examples of this include requiring managed care organizations to provide screening and referral services to address SDoH as seen in Wisconsin, embedding community health worker interventions delivered by culturally and linguistically competent community-based organizations (CBOs) as in Michigan, and collecting data on the housing needs of beneficiaries in Tennessee (ASTHO, 2022).

- Use accountable care organization models to assign providers responsibility for the costs and quality of a defined community's health.
- Align policies across state health insurance programs like Medicaid, the Children's Health Insurance Program (CHIP), and state employee insurance, as well as between state insurance programs and state social service entities to better support health outcomes. This alignment could be achieved by standardizing the data collected and eliminating barriers to interagency data sharing to identify gaps in access and track receipt of health-related services and supports across community settings.
- Require that all nonprofit hospitals (those hospitals receiving tax exemptions, as described in footnote 3) engage in multi-stakeholder collaborations to establish and finance locally controlled pools of funds with a neutral community entity as a fiscal agent similar to the Massachusetts Prevention & Wellness Trust Fund program (MPHA, 2019). The fund would create a sustainable mechanism for combining—either through braiding or blending[1]—financial resources from different sources to build and sustain community infrastructure (Urban Institute, 2022). Goals might include:
  —50 percent of community collaborations (such as Accountable Communities for Health) establishing a locally controlled pool of funds, which would be governed by consumer-led advisory councils in 2030. This pool of funds would enable communities to make community-based decisions on allocating resources toward building and sustaining access to community-based interventions, infrastructure, and capacity building;
  —50 percent of community collaborations with locally controlled pools of funds allocating sufficient funding for community infrastructure by 2030;
  —50 percent of communities developing social service networks consisting of CBOs and entities. The network would specialize in providing services that address needs identified in community health needs assessments (CHNAs) and community health assessments (CHAs) by 2030; and
  —50 percent of nonprofit hospitals in each state contributing to locally controlled community funds by 2030 to ensure more health financing is controlled by communities. The amount donated would be the difference between reported charity care as a percent of operating expenses in the

---

[1] Blended and braided funding involves combining two or more sources of funding toward a program or activity. Braided funding pools funding streams toward a single purpose while accounting, tracking, and reporting for each funding source. Unlike braided funding, blended funding does not account, track, or report for each funding source. These strategies can be used to attract limited financing from more than one source to fund needed public policy priorities. However, effectively braiding funding streams requires organizations to track requirements, metrics, and measures of different funders.

current fiscal year and the charity care average of the past 3 years as a percentage of operating expenses.
- Design and require the use of Health Impact Assessments (HIAs)—like Environmental Impact Assessments (EIAs)[2]—to assess the impact of policy proposals and business activities on health, particularly in sectors where health impacts may not be currently considered (Cole and Fielding, 2007). HIAs could be applied to the creation of new policies, projects, and programs or the implementation of existing ones. HIAs can also inform EIAs, which often do not consider health outcomes. Mandatory HIAs would not force decision-makers to act on the information but would ensure awareness and consideration of the potential health effects when considering programmatic and policy decisions.
- Develop, or require the development of, cross-sector data sharing capabilities to facilitate cross-platform collaboration between public health, insurance, social services, and care delivery information systems. Health information exchanges, all payer claims databases, and social services referral networks are all examples of data aggregators that are not currently integrated in utilizing their data toward realizing whole person, whole population health in an aligned fashion.

Incremental and Intermediate Action

- Require nonprofit health systems to apply community benefit dollars[3] toward impact investments that improve social, economic, and environmental conditions in disadvantaged communities while also producing economic returns for investors. Considering that for-profit hospitals in aggregate provided more charity care than nonprofit hospitals per every $100 in total expenses, this action would require the benefits of tax exemptions and subsidies to be passed onto the community (Hyman and Bai, 2022).

---

[2] An Environmental Impact Assessment evaluates the environmental consequences of a policy, plan, or project before a decision to move forward is made. It requires decision-makers to consider environmental values in their decisions and to justify those decisions should they decide to implement a plan.

[3] Almost 70 percent of U.S. hospitals are not-for-profit entities and are therefore exempt from federal, state, and local taxes in recognition of their "community benefit." Community benefit refers to the activities undertaken by these hospitals to improve the health of the communities they serve. The Affordable Care Act (ACA) added a section to the IRS code that contained new requirements related to community benefits that nonprofit hospitals must meet to qualify for tax-exempt status. These requirements include conducting a CHNA and having a written financial assistance policy for medically necessary and emergency care.

The following table provides an overview of the Steering Group's judgment of the impact and feasibility of the priority actions described above.

Priority Action	Category	Impact Rating (1 to 5) 1-least impactful; 5-most impactful	Feasibility Rating (1 to 5) 1-least feasible; 5-most feasible
Pursue and use 1115 waivers to cover innovative care and payment models that address social determinants of health.	Transformative	3.6	4
Require managed care organizations to focus on prevention and social determinants of health through Medicaid managed care contracts.	Transformative	3.4	4
Use accountable care organization models to assign providers responsibility for the costs and quality of a defined community's health.	Transformative	3.4	3
Align policies across state health insurance programs like Medicaid, Children's Health Insurance Program, and state employee insurance, as well as between state insurance programs and state social service entities to better support health outcomes.	Transformative	3.4	2.8
Require that all nonprofit hospitals engage in multi-stakeholder collaborations to establish and finance locally controlled pools of funds with a neutral community entity as a fiscal agent similar to the Massachusetts Prevention & Wellness Trust Fund program.	Transformative	4.6	3.2
Design and require the use of HIAs to assess the impact of policy proposals and business activities on health, particularly in sectors where health impacts may not be currently considered.	Transformative	3.4	3.4
Develop, or require the development of, cross-sector, data-sharing capabilities to facilitate cross-platform collaboration between public health, insurance, social services, and care delivery information systems.	Transformative	3.4	2.6

Require nonprofit health systems to apply community benefit dollars toward impact investments that improve social, economic, and environmental conditions in disadvantaged communities while also producing economic returns for investors.	Intermediate and Incremental	3.3	3.8

Community Benefit Oversight. Nonprofit hospitals comprise about 70 percent of all hospitals in the United States. These hospitals are exempt from federal, state, and local taxes because they meet requirements to provide charity care and other benefits to the community in which they operate (CAP, 2022). However, the U.S. Internal Revenue Code requirements for nonprofit hospitals are relatively general and do not specify a minimum value or type of community benefits that must be provided to receive this exemption. States have the authority to strengthen, clarify, and expand these requirements in service of whole person and population health (CAP, 2022).

Transformative Actions

- Set performance goals to improve health outcomes and transform nonprofit hospitals' approaches to consumer engagement and care. Key goals to achieve by 2030 could include:
  - —50 percent of nonprofit hospitals' CHNAs and community health improvement plans (CHIPs) involve developing and/or engaging in cross-sector collaborations (such as local or regional accountable communities for health) that include consumers in at least 10 percent of activities;
  - —50 percent of CHNAs and CHIPs reported each year specify the dollar amounts necessary to build effective cross-sector collaborations or sustain those already in existence;
  - —50 percent of reporting entities' community benefit investments emphasize or catalyze cross-sector collaborations aligned with priorities identified in local CHNAs and CHIPs; and
  - —50 percent of cross-sector collaborations formed by reporting entities are community-governed, with at least 20 percent authentic representation of consumers with lived experiences.

Intermediate and Incremental Actions

- Amplify baseline federal requirements to promote meaningful engagement of cross-sector and/or community-governed collaborations in nonprofit hospitals' CHNAs and public health departments' CHAs. For example, by engaging community actors in assessing health and social service providers' capacity as part of the needs assessment process, hospitals and public health departments can look beyond programming focused largely on addressing health conditions toward strengthening community infrastructure to improve wellness more broadly.

- Require the standardization and integration of CHNAs conducted by hospitals within the same health system to yield robust data on unmet health and health-related social needs within a designated service area. The data can then be shared across hospitals and with other community actors to inform system- and community-wide programs to address unmet needs across institutions and local jurisdictions.
- Leverage state authority to make appointments to the boards of public hospitals that ensure meaningful community representation. Require nonprofit hospitals to do the same, as a condition of their tax exemption.
- Use certificate of need decisions to address inequities and disparities relating to access to primary care, geographic location, race, ethnicity, disability status, etc.

The following table provides an overview of the Steering Group's judgment of the impact and feasibility of the priority actions described above.

Priority Action	Category	Impact Rating (1 to 5) 1-least impactful; 5-most impactful	Feasibility Rating (1 to 5) 1-least feasible; 5-most feasible
Set performance goals to improve health outcomes and transform nonprofit hospitals' approaches to consumer engagement and care.	Transformative	3.8	3
Amplify baseline federal requirements to promote meaningful engagement of cross-sector and/or community-governed collaborations as key components in CHNAs and CHAs.	Intermediate and Incremental	2.6	3.2
Require the standardization and integration of CHNAs conducted by hospitals within the same health system to yield robust data on unmet health and health-related social needs within a designated service area.	Intermediate and Incremental	2.4	3.8

| Leverage state authority to make appointments to the boards of public hospitals that ensure meaningful community representation. | Intermediate and Incremental | 2 | 3.8 |
| Use certificate of need decisions to address inequities and disparities relating to access to primary care, geographic location, race, ethnicity, disability status, etc. | Intermediate and Incremental | 3 | 3.2 |

Insurance Oversight. States have the vantage point to see the health system as a whole in ways that individual providers, payers, patients, and even communities do not, putting them in the position to shape health payment systems through legislation and regulation of commercial payers selling plans to state employers and residents.

Transformative Actions

- Adopt and expand laws and regulations pertaining to health insurance rate review[4] and, specifically approval authority. Use that authority to accelerate payer reform, alignment, and whole person and population health. Regulatory targets could include:
  —Incorporate considerations around affordability and access, particularly for high-value primary care, into rate review criteria.
  —Require disclosures of data on the health status of covered populations, including stratification across factors such as but not limited to race, ethnicity, geographic location, and income.
  —Require the creation and implementation of equity plans to ensure that rate increases do not contribute to disparities in affordability and access. A component of this plan should be an assessment of coordination between in-network health systems and community-based organizations to evaluate access to health-related services such as food, housing, and transportation.

Intermediate and Incremental Action

- Leverage state insurance department approval processes to institute usual source of care requirements for fully insured health plans. These requirements could include screening and referral of enrollees to a usual source of care and educating program staff on usual source of care benefits. Requiring a usual

---

[4] Health insurance rate review is a process "designed to improve insurer accountability and transparency [by evaluating] whether insurers' proposed annual rate increases are based on reasonable cost assumptions and solid evidence and [allowing] consumers the chance to comment on proposed increases." See https://ratereview.healthcare.gov (accessed October 5, 2022).

source of care in health plans will increase care coordination across behavioral, oral, primary care, and specialty services, thereby improving health outcomes.

The following table provides an overview of the Steering Group's judgment of the impact and feasibility of the priority actions described above.

Priority Action	Category	Impact Rating (1 to 5) 1-least impactful; 5-most impactful	Feasibility Rating (1 to 5) 1-least feasible; 5-most feasible
Adopt and expand laws and regulations pertaining to health insurance rate review and, specifically, approval authority.	Transformative	4.2	3.2
Leverage state insurance department approval processes to institute usual source of care requirements for fully insured health plans.	Intermediate and Incremental	3	3.3

Appropriations. States also have the authority to appropriate and allocate funding toward policies, programs, and services that support whole person and population health, including education, public welfare, health care, infrastructure, legal services, and housing and community development initiatives. Allocation of resources with the goal of improving health would require states to consider and apply a health-in-all-policies approach.

Transformative Action

- Place unspent government funds from pandemic-era legislation such as the American Rescue Plan Act into community-governed pools and allow service beneficiaries and navigators to govern their use toward upstream determinants of health and social services. State dental funding in Hawaii and pooled HIV funding in New York are examples of this approach.

Intermediate and Incremental Action

- Earmark funds for structured training at the local level to strengthen political and health literacy, as well as civic engagement and community governance skills. New Orleans, Louisiana, and Charlotte, North Carolina, are two examples of cities that provide free training to help residents build the necessary skills to improve quality of life in their communities.

The following table provides an overview of the Steering Group's judgment of the impact and feasibility of the priority actions described above.

Priority Action	Category	Impact Rating (1 to 5) 1-least impactful; 5-most impactful	Feasibility Rating (1 to 5) 1-least feasible; 5-most feasible
Place unspent government funds from pandemic-era legislation such as the American Rescue Plan Act into community-governed pools and allow service beneficiaries and navigators to govern their use toward upstream determinants of health and social services.	Transformative	3.6	2.8
Earmark funds for structured training at the local level to strengthen political and health literacy, as well as civic engagement and community governance skills.	Intermediate and Incremental	2.8	3.4

Public Health Agencies and Departments. As discussed in Chapters 1 and 2, public health agencies at all levels of government have been chronically underfunded and underserved, limiting the impact they can have on the communities they serve. Responsible for health promotion and disease prevention, public health agencies are well suited to serve as backbone organizations of multi-stakeholder coalitions to address whole health issues at the local and state levels if properly resourced.

Transformational Actions

- Provided the necessary resources, lead the development of community-wide goals and collective impact strategies to improve health and equity, involving multiple government agencies, nonprofit partners, and the private sector. Support the full engagement of community residents in the process.
- Partner with health care organizations incentivized to better health outcomes to codevelop and lead community programs that advance prevention. Support the full engagement of community residents and local organizations in the process.

Intermediate and Incremental Actions

- Lead coordination of CHAs and CHNAs, so that they provide opportunities for meaningful engagement of community residents, address key determinants

of health, and advance prevention across the community, shifting collective emphasis away from individual conditions (such as diabetes and heart disease) to community infrastructure that better supports health.
- Create protocols for systematically assessing the capacity of community health and social service providers to determine how the community as a whole can address service gaps in an efficient, collective, and sustainable way.
- Utilize public health authority as appropriate to allow community-supported strategies to have the greatest impact. For example, if a goal is to reduce falls among the elderly, the health department can receive reports of emergency department visits to identify areas of a community in need of additional resources.

The following table provides an overview of the Steering Group's judgment of the impact and feasibility of the priority actions described above.

Priority Action	Category	Impact Rating (1 to 5) 1-least impactful; 5-most impactful	Feasibility Rating (1 to 5) 1-least feasible; 5-most feasible
Lead the development of community-wide goals and collective impact strategies to improve health and equity, involving multiple government agencies, nonprofit partners, and the private sector. Support the full engagement of community residents in the process.	Transformative	4	2.4
Partner with health care organizations incentivized to better health outcomes to codevelop and lead community programs that advance prevention. Support the full engagement of community residents and local organizations in the process.	Transformative	4	3.8
Lead coordination of CHAs and CHNAs, so that they provide opportunities for meaningful engagement of community residents, address key determinants of health, and advance prevention across the community, shifting collective emphasis away from individual conditions (such as diabetes and heart disease) to community infrastructure that better supports health.	Intermediate and Incremental	3.2	3.4

Create protocols for systematically assessing the capacity of community health and social service providers to determine how the community as a whole can address service gaps in an efficient, collective, and sustainable way.	Intermediate and Incremental	2.4	3.6
Utilize public health authority as appropriate to allow community-supported strategies to have the greatest impact.	Intermediate and Incremental	2.5	2.3

Federal Government

The legislative and executive branches of the U.S. federal government are vested with the power to make new laws or change existing laws and implement or enforce laws passed by Congress, respectively. Where aligned, these two branches of the federal government (the legislative and executive) have substantial latitude to legislate and enforce landmark laws such as the Medicare and Medicaid Act or the Patient Protection and Affordable Care Act (ACA). Given the political will, the federal government could leverage its broad authority to significantly advance additional health-promoting policies and appropriate more resources to support the implementation of health-supporting programs (The White House, 2022a,b).

Transformative Actions

- Expand ACA requirements governing "essential benefits" for plans sold in the individual and small group markets. Added supports and services could include integrative care, home- and community-based services, and caregiver services.[5]
- Review Employee Retirement Income Security Act of 1974 (ERISA) and large group insurance requirements to add integrative care and home and community services and supports as essential benefits.

---

[5] The ACA requires health plans in small and individual group markets to cover essential health benefits, which include services in 10 benefit categories: ambulatory patient services; emergency services; hospitalization; maternity and newborn care; mental health and substance use disorder services, including behavioral health treatment; prescription drugs; rehabilitative and habilitative services and devices; laboratory services; preventive and wellness services and chronic disease management; and pediatric services, including oral and vision care. While these essential health benefits reflect comprehensive coverage of health care services, they do not include many services that have been shown to improve health. Expanding this definition of essential health benefits for small group and individual insurance plans to encompass integrative care, home- and community-based services, and caregiver services as appropriate would go far in ensuring people are connected with support to maintain and advance whole health.

- Revise the medical loss ratios (MLRs) used in the ACA to become "health loss ratios" that support health rather than health care. The MLR is a financial metric to ensure health plans provide value to enrollees by spending 80 percent or more of their premium income on health care claims and quality improvement (as opposed to administration, marketing, and profit). A health loss ratio would require plans to spend a certain percentage of their premium income not only on paying medical claims but on proven investments to maintain and improve their enrollees' health, providing flexibility for health plans and, by extension, health service providers to invest in more non–health care related social drivers and community resources.
- Design and require the use of health impact assessments (HIAs)—like environmental impact assessments (EIAs)[6]—to assess the impact of policy proposals and business activities on health, particularly in sectors where health impacts may not be currently considered (Cole and Fielding, 2007). HIAs could be applied to the creation of new policies, projects, and programs or the implementation of existing ones. HIAs can also inform EIAs, which often do not consider health outcomes. Mandatory HIAs would not force decision-makers to act on the information but would ensure awareness and consideration of the potential health effects when considering programmatic and policy decisions.
- Supplement federal health care reform efforts to create a federal benefits package that incentivizes an expanded or reconsidered set of "essential benefits" (e.g., home- and community-based services [HCBS], "in lieu of" services).
- Require that all nonprofit hospitals engage in multi-stakeholder collaborations to establish and finance locally controlled pools of funds with a neutral community entity as a fiscal agent similar to the Massachusetts Prevention & Wellness Trust Fund program (MPHA, 2019). The fund would create a sustainable funding mechanism for combining—either through braiding or blending[7]—financial resources from different sources to build and sustain community infrastructure (Urban Institute, 2022). Goals might include:

---

[6] An environmental impact assessment evaluates the environmental consequences of a policy, plan, or project before a decision to move forward is made. It requires decision-makers to consider environmental values in their decisions and to justify those decisions should they decide to implement a plan.

[7] Blended and braided funding involves combining two or more sources of funding toward a program or activity. Braided funding pools funding streams toward a single purpose while accounting, tracking, and reporting for each funding source. Unlike braided funding, blended funding does not account, track, or report for each funding source. These strategies can be used to attract limited financing from more than one source to fund needed public policy priorities. However, effectively braiding funding streams requires organizations to track requirements, metrics, and measures of different funders.

—50 percent of community collaborations (such as accountable communities for health) establishing a locally controlled pool of funds, which would be governed by consumer-led advisory councils in 2030. This pool of funds would enable communities to make community-based decisions on allocating resources toward building and sustaining access to community-based interventions, infrastructure, and capacity-building;

—50 percent of community collaborations with locally controlled pools of funds allocating sufficient funding for community infrastructure by 2030;

—50 percent of communities developing social service networks consisting of CBOs and entities. The network would specialize in providing services that address needs identified in CHNAs and CHAs by 2030; and

—50 percent of nonprofit hospitals in each state contributing to locally controlled community funds by 2030 to ensure more health financing is controlled by communities. The amount donated would be the difference between reported charity care as a percent of operating expenses in the current fiscal year and the charity care average of the past 3 years as a percentage of operating expenses.

- Require nonprofit hospitals and health systems to apply community benefit dollars[8] toward impact investments that improve social, economic, and environmental conditions in disadvantaged communities while also producing economic returns for investors. Considering that for-profit hospitals in aggregate provided more charity care than nonprofit hospitals per every $100 in total expenses, this action would require the benefits of tax exemptions and subsidies to be passed onto the community (Hyman and Bai, 2022).

- Create a parsimonious set of performance measures that provide meaningful information on the most important outcomes at the individual and community levels. An important model in this respect is presented in the 2015 Institute of Medicine report *Vital Signs: Core Metrics for Health and Health Care Progress*. These measures could be created by building off *Vital Signs* measures, and the related work of the Centers for Medicare & Medicaid Services (CMS) on Medicaid HCBS, as well as for Medicare-Medicaid enrollees in its Meaningful Measures initiative. These measures would be whole person (i.e., not focused on one diagnosis or a narrow set of clinical experiences) and inclusive of an

---

[8] Almost 70 percent of U.S. hospitals are not-for-profit entities and are therefore exempt from federal, state, and local taxes in recognition of their "community benefit." Community benefit refers to the activities undertaken by these hospitals to improve the health of the communities they serve. The ACA added a section to the IRS code that contained new requirements related to community benefits that nonprofit hospitals must meet to qualify for tax-exempt status. These requirements include conducting a CHNA and having a written financial assistance policy for medically necessary and emergency care.

individual's nonclinical needs, preferences, and goals for enhanced health and well-being in ways that matter to the individual. In addition, the measures should be stratified across race, ethnicity, income, and disability to ensure a focus on monitoring and targeting inequities and implicit bias in measure sets.
- Require a 2 to 5 percent withholding from current federal grants to state programs to create a flexible federally funded pool for which localities or states could apply to implement community-governed whole person health improvement strategies. Eligibility would be provided to communities with the worst health outcomes and applicants would include a wide array of participants across the care and services continuum with an aligned governing structure and strategic plan. This funding pool would employ flexible federal requirements across programs that waive existing and conflicting program rules; optimize existing funds to support regional or local whole health interventions; offer tax credits and subsidies for entities that meaningfully participate with funding from the pool; and would require that earned interest be used for social service alignment.
- CMS should stop paying for interventions or services not proven to improve health outcomes (such as low-value care identified by the Choosing Wisely campaign) in the vein of CMS's 2008 rule ending reimbursement for hospital-acquired conditions. CMS should also increase scrutiny of new and existing therapeutics and adjust their reimbursement policies accordingly, following the example of a 2022 rule requiring Medicare Part D sponsors to establish drug management programs for beneficiaries who are at risk for misuse or abuse of opioids.

Intermediate and Incremental Actions

- Create a funding pool modeled off the CMMI State Innovation Model (SIM) that would incentivize less-resourced states or regions to adopt population-based global budgets, specifically focusing on improving children's health,[9] as communities, health care payers, and providers often need financial support to transition to innovative payment models that support whole person care (e.g.,

---

[9] A new SIM grant focused on children's health would yield long-term returns on population health (NASEM, 2021). In the past, it has been challenging to justify investments in pediatric health models due to a narrow 3- to 5-year time horizon for measuring returns on investment under the typical performance period for Center for Medicare & Medicaid Innovation models (Podulka and Narayan, 2021). However, with a longer-term focus, investments in children's health would be easier to defend from a financial perspective. This challenge underscores the need to lengthen the time frame for calculating and evaluating actuarial return on investment.

all-payer global budgets).[10] For example, Pennsylvania received $25 million from CMS to provide technical assistance and other support through its new Rural Health Redesign Center.
- Increase funding and support for programs that address health-related social factors. Other sources of funding include private philanthropy, foundations, and the global budgets themselves, which can be set up to provide additional room for population health investments (Sharfstein et al., 2017). These programs could be supported in part by providing flexibility and guidance to stakeholders with respect to better unifying federally funded programs across a whole-of-government framework on whole person health and well-being. A focus on whole health would enable the government to fill the gaps between federally funded programs across the U.S. Department of Education (Individualized Education Programs), the U.S. Department of Agriculture (Supplemental Nutrition Assistance Program and National School Lunch Program), the U.S. Department of Health and Human Services (Temporary Assistance for Needy Families, Federally Qualified Health Centers, and Medicaid), the U.S. Department of Labor (workforce development programs), and others. By filling these gaps, the integration of these programs would result in a comprehensive suite of population-based health services and supports. Financial incentives could also be provided to drive collaboration and alignment between Medicaid and social service programs at the state level.
- Create a commission to deliver recommendations to Congress on how to restructure existing health and social service programs to bring greater value to consumers and taxpayers.
- Strengthen and optimize Community Health Needs Assessments to center on community-governed interventions and funding in order to enhance collective financing mechanisms listed in the previous section.
- Pioneer the development and implementation of payment models based on priorities of community-based organizations and designed with their partnership. These payment models would reward health systems for contributing to community health and well-being improvements.

The following table provides an overview of the Steering Group's judgment of the impact and feasibility of the priority actions described above.

---

[10] A National Academies' committee recently noted, "Even when there is financial alignment, organizations with fewer resources may not be able to respond ... without upfront resources" (NASEM, 2016).

Priority Action	Category	Impact Rating (1 to 5) 1-least impactful; 5-most impactful	Feasibility Rating (1 to 5) 1-least feasible; 5-most feasible
Expand ACA requirements governing "essential benefits" for plans sold in the individual and small group markets.	Transformative	4.2	2.8
Review ERISA and large group insurance requirements to add integrative care and home and community services and supports as essential benefits.	Transformative	3.6	2.6
Revise the medical loss ratios used in the ACA to become "health loss ratios" that support health rather than health care.	Transformative	4.4	3.0
Design and require the use of health impact assessments to assess the impact of policy proposals and business activities on health, particularly in sectors where health impacts may not be currently considered.	Transformative	3.8	2.8
Supplement federal health care reform efforts to create a federal benefits package that incentivizes an expanded or reconsidered set of "essential benefits."	Transformative	4	2.8
Require that all nonprofit hospitals engage in multi-stakeholder collaborations to establish and finance locally controlled pools of funds with a neutral community entity as a fiscal agent.	Transformative	3.8	2.4
Require nonprofit health systems to apply community benefit dollars toward impact investments that improve social, economic, and environmental conditions in disadvantaged communities.	Transformative	3.4	3.4
Create a parsimonious set of quality measures that provide meaningful information on person-centered health and well-being outcomes.	Transformative	3.6	4.4
Require a 2% to 5% withholding from current federal grants to state programs to create a flexible federally funded pool for which localities or states could apply to implement community-governed whole person health improvement strategies.	Transformative	3.6	3.2

CMS should stop paying for interventions or services not proven to improve health outcomes and increase scrutiny of new and existing therapeutics, adjusting their reimbursement policies accordingly.	Transformative	3.4	3.2
Create a funding pool modeled off the CMMI State Innovation Model that would incentivize less-resourced states or regions to adopt population-based global budgets, specifically focusing on improving children's health, as communities, health care payers, and providers often need financial support to transition to innovative payment models that support whole person care (e.g., all-payer global budgets).	Intermediate and Incremental	2.8	3.4
Increase funding and support for programs that address health-related social factors.	Intermediate and Incremental	3.0	2.6
Create a commission to deliver recommendations to Congress on how to restructure existing health and social service programs to bring greater value to consumers and taxpayers.	Intermediate and Incremental	2.0	4.4
Strengthen and optimize CHNAs to center on community-governed interventions and funding in order to enhance collective financing mechanisms listed in the previous section.	Intermediate and Incremental	3.2	3.8
Pioneer the development and implementation of payment models based on priorities of CBOs and designed with their partnership.	Intermediate and Incremental	3.2	3.2

Examples of how federal government policy changes, actions, and communications can influence a multisector cascade of change, including in state and local governments as well as the financial sector, are detailed in Appendix C.

Care Delivery Organizations and Health Systems

Comprising more than 15 percent of the U.S. economy and standing at the front lines of health care, care delivery organizations, including hospitals and health systems, play a vital role in ensuring the health of patients, families, and communities. To ensure these organizations most efficiently, effectively, and equitably foster whole health, incentives must be restructured to reduce the financial benefits of volume-dependent care and increase the attractiveness of value-based models that incorporate community health workers and other health professionals. Financial incentives must also be directed toward public health, especially social drivers of whole person, whole population health. Moreover, whole ecosystems adjacent to health systems, including information technology infrastructure, schools, and the legal system, must be meaningfully engaged to build the necessary upstream conditions to ensure the key tenets of whole person, whole population health, which include human thriving, sharing data to improve care quality, and targeting population-specific health issues.

Transformative Actions

- Transform the landscape of economic incentives to support whole person health by transitioning 75 percent of the health system reimbursement framework to population-based payments.
- Pursue multilevel approaches to working collaboratively with community stakeholders, such as:
  — Fair compensation for community health workers;
  — Credibly and meaningfully integrating community voices into health system strategy and decision-making; and
  — Building meaningful alliances with a broad ecosystem of CBOs like social services, food and nutrition experts, behavioral health experts, and substance use experts, in addition to law enforcement, emergency response, criminal justice, and schools.
- Invest in information technology infrastructure that can catalyze gains in community health, such as robust information exchange and data-sharing processes between care delivery organizations and CBOs, as well as "digital front doors" (i.e., health kiosks) in the community. Where technology is used by the public, these services should also reduce the digital divide through reduced barriers to access, education on technology navigation and use, and the availability of nontechnological alternatives.
- Screen patients for health-related social needs—such as access to food, shelter, and transportation—and provide closed-loop referrals via community information exchanges to social service entities and community-based organizations that can meet those needs.

Intermediate and Incremental Actions

- Set goals for an increased amount of community benefit dollars and grants spent on evidence-based services and strategies that strengthen whole person, population health and well-being (e.g., public transportation services, nutritious meals programs, and stable housing initiatives).

- Align the compensation structure of senior executives to health system performance on a set of community defined health metrics.
- Establish a community liaison infrastructure within the health system to align activities and create shared expectations with CBOs.

The following table provides an overview of the Steering Group's judgment of the impact and feasibility of the priority actions described above.

Priority Action	Category	Impact Rating (1 to 5) *1-least impactful; 5-most impactful*	Feasibility Rating (1 to 5) *1-least feasible; 5-most feasible*
Transform the landscape of economic incentives to support whole person health by transitioning 75% of the health system reimbursement framework to population-based payments.	Transformative	4.6	2.2
Pursue multilevel approaches to working collaboratively with community stakeholders, such as fair compensation for community health workers, credibly and meaningfully integrating community voices into health system strategy and decision-making, and building meaningful alliances with a broad ecosystem of community organizations.	Transformative	3.8	2.6
Invest in information technology infrastructure that can catalyze gains in community health, such as robust information exchange and data-sharing processes between care delivery organizations and CBOs, as well as "digital front doors" (i.e., health kiosks) in the community.	Transformative	3.4	3.4
Screen patients for social determinants of health and health-related social needs and provide closed-loop referrals to social service entities and CBOs that can meet those needs.	Transformative	4.2	4.5
Set goals for an increased amount of community benefit dollars and grants spent on evidence-based services and strategies that strengthen whole person, whole population health and well-being.	Intermediate and Incremental	3.2	3.6

Align the compensation structure of senior executives to health system performance on a set of community defined health metrics.	Intermediate and Incremental	3.2	2.2
Establish a community liaison infrastructure within the health system to align activities and create shared expectations with CBOs.	Intermediate and Incremental	2.8	3.4

Payers

By negotiating rates for provider services and setting premium and deductible rates for consumers, private and public payers control key financial levers needed to transform care delivery (Brookings Health System, 2022). As a result, payers' negotiation, contracting, and other business practices have tremendous power to cultivate whole person, whole population health.

Transformative Actions

- Establish processes to routinely identify the social needs of health plan members and direct investments toward resources to address those needs. Engage entities such as the United Way, CMMI, CMS network lead entities, and others that are either large payers or entities that can credibly convene authentic and diverse community voices (churches, youth groups, school associations, etc.) to surface member needs and priorities.
- Create a population health business model where private payers such as commercial health insurance plans, insurance plan providers, health systems, and, if possible, CMS pay CBOs to create value and improve health and well-being by facilitating healthy opportunities.
- Evaluate and expand on the scope of "essential benefits" (e.g., HCBS, "in lieu of" services) required under the ACA to include guaranteed coverage for services that produce whole health and well-being.
- Reimburse care delivery organizations, social service entities, and community-based organizations for closed-loop referrals targeting member social determinants of health and health-related social needs.
- Hold health systems accountable to anchor organization[11] practices that will promote whole person, whole population health through payer-provider contracts. Examples of these practices include the Anchor Mission approach, which encourages hospitals and universities to create pipelines for local community members to obtain employment and upward mobility within

---

[11] Anchor institutions are nonprofit or public place-based entities such as universities and hospitals that are rooted in their community through mission, invested capital, or relationships to customers, employees, residents, and vendors.

anchor organizations; procure services through local businesses; utilize available cash reserves toward long-term community projects that will enhance sustainability and inclusion; and utilize grants or impact investing to develop affordable housing. These practices also provide opportunities to impact key health system issues such as the fair compensation for community health workers or the need to include historically and/or presently marginalized communities in organizational decisions. Hospitals such as Bon Secours Mercy Health in Ohio and the Richmond University Medical Center in Virginia have implemented elements of this approach.

Intermediate and Incremental Actions

- Pioneer the development and implementation of payment models based on priorities of community-based organizations and designed with their partnership. These payment models would reward health systems for contributing to community health and well-being improvements.
- Build alliances with key community partners (e.g., law enforcement, emergency response, criminal justice, schools, and social services providers) that encourage cooperation within the local ecosystem to support outcomes aligned with the Quintuple Aim. Examples include the BUILD Health Challenge Model and the Washington State Accountable Communities of Health.
- Reduce practice consolidation by implementing payment policies inclusive of small, independent health care practices. This strategy would involve aggregate[12] practices across specialties and functions in aggregate entities that are less formally integrated than managed services organizations.

The following table provides an overview of the Steering Group's judgment of the impact and feasibility of the priority actions described above.

---

[12] Aggregation can be defined as the *partial* linking of distinct units. These units can include hospitals, practices, claims, electronic health records (EHRs), or any other component within the health care system (Liaw et al., 2017).

Priority Action	Category	Impact Rating (1 to 5) 1-least impactful; 5-most impactful	Feasibility Rating (1 to 5) 1-least feasible; 5-most feasible
Establish processes to routinely identify the social needs of the health plan members and direct investments toward resources to address those needs.	Transformative	4.3	4.4
Create a population health business model where private payers such as commercial health insurance plans, insurance plan providers, health systems, and, if possible, CMS pay CBOs to create value and improve health and well-being by facilitating healthy opportunities.	Transformative	4.4	3.4
Evaluate and expand on the scope of "essential benefits" required under the ACA to include guaranteed coverage for services that produce whole health and well-being.	Transformative	3.8	3.2
Reimburse care delivery organizations, social service entities, and community-based organizations for closed-loop referrals targeting member social determinants of health and health-related social needs.	Transformative	3.4	3.2
Hold health systems accountable to anchor organization practices that will promote whole person, whole population health through payer-provider contracts.	Transformative	3.8	2.0
Pioneer the development and implementation of payment models based on priorities of CBOs and designed with their partnership.	Intermediate and Incremental	3.2	3.2
Build alliances with key community partners (e.g., law enforcement, emergency response, criminal justice, schools, and social services providers) that encourage cooperation within the local ecosystem to support outcomes aligned with the Quintuple Aim.	Intermediate and Incremental	3.2	4.0
Reduce practice consolidation by implementing payment policies inclusive of small, independent health care practices.	Intermediate and Incremental	2.8	4.0

Employers

Employers from all sectors collectively employ more than 164 million people in the United States. Through the work environments they foster and the benefits they offer, employers play a significant role in shaping the health of their employees, as well as others in their communities (BLS, 2022). In addition to creating healthy work environments and providing leadership on community health issues, employers can use their significant collective economic clout to advance employee-driven population health initiatives and negotiate with providers to accelerate the routine delivery of whole person care.

Transformative Actions

- Enhance workforce well-being by establishing an expanded set of "essential benefits" in health benefit packages provided to employees that includes relevant social services (see federal government section for additional detail).
- Establish linkages and partnerships with health care, local government, CBOs, and philanthropies that leverage employers' position as community cornerstones, which includes:
  —their ability to influence individual employees within and outside the workplace,
  —their power as purchasers of health plans, and
  —the impact of their businesses on the local environment.
- Join forces to apply employers' collective economic power in their communities to address health-related social challenges impacting members of the community, including employees. An example of one such partnership is the NOLA Coalition, which aims to harness members' collective resources to create a safer and more prosperous New Orleans through near-term actions to reduce violence, in addition to a 3-year, $15 million program that aims to strengthen social services to support youth and drive generational change (NOLA Coalition, 2022).

Intermediate and Incremental Actions

- Capitalize on sector market power to purchase health plans that provide access to closed-loop referrals that target members' health-related social needs, including access to food, shelter, and transportation.
- Set minimum expectations for how health plans should contract and collaborate with community-based organizations.
- Incentivize employees through employer-purchased health plans to seek care from in-network practitioners with expertise in health behavior change, healthy lifestyles, and wellness (e.g., lifestyle medicine, integrative medicine).

The following table provides an overview of the Steering Group's judgment of the impact and feasibility of the priority actions described above.

Priority Action	Category	Impact Rating (1 to 5) 1–least impactful; 5–most impactful	Feasibility Rating (1 to 5) 1–least feasible; 5–most feasible
Enhance workforce well-being by establishing an expanded set of "essential benefits" in health benefit packages provided to employees that includes relevant social services.	Transformative	4.0	3.8
Establish linkages and partnerships with health care, local government, CBOs, and philanthropies that leverage employers' position as community cornerstones, which includes: their ability to influence individual employees within and outside the workplace; their power as purchasers of health plans; and the impact of their businesses on the local environment.	Transformative	3.4	3.6
Join forces to apply employers' collective economic power in their communities to address health-related social challenges impacting members of the community, including employees.	Transformative	3.4	3.0
Capitalize on sector market power to purchase health plans that provide access to closed-loop referrals that target members' health-related social needs.	Intermediate and Incremental	3.3	3.5
Set minimum expectations for how health plans should contract and collaborate with CBOs.	Intermediate and Incremental	2.6	2.6
Incentivize employees through employer-purchased health plans to seek care from in-network practitioners with expertise in health behavior change, healthy lifestyles, and wellness (e.g., lifestyle medicine, integrative medicine).	Intermediate and Incremental	2.8	2.6

Financial Sector Organizations

As of September 30, 2022, the total market capitalization of the U.S. stock market was around $46 trillion, with capital invested in 11 sectors of publicly listed companies, including but not limited to health care, financials, real estate, consumer staples, and energy (MSCI, 2022; Siblis Research, 2022). The substantial overlap and market power of these companies provide a significant opportunity to reshape markets to incentivize and reward whole person, whole population health. The following are opportunities for action for finance leaders both within and beyond the health care sector that would significantly impact how health is valued and financed. These stakeholders include chief financial officers of corporations, investment units within banking institutions, and leaders of venture capital/private equity firms.

Transformative Actions

- Create industry and professional standards (e.g., for hospitals, health plan actuaries, and chief financial officers at all health care organizations) that redefine return on investment (ROI) in a way that explicitly quantifies the economic value of health in the population being served. Consider the business case for financial returns derived from economic productivity driven by better workforce and community health.
- In tandem with the right regulatory incentives, forge partnerships with a diverse array of entities to ensure that financing sources correspond with the entities that benefit from services in terms of ROI. For example, if an asthma remediation effort reduces employee absenteeism (because working parents less frequently have to stay home with asthmatic children), employers should contribute toward the cost of the remediation effort in the community. In forging these partnerships, financial sector organizations should consider the following:
  —Benefits and their impact across sectors must be captured, defined, and measured.
  —Subsidies might be necessary if the sum of the benefits, properly mapped to various nongovernmental stakeholders, does not equal the cost of the intervention, as benefits would also accrue to the public sector (e.g., in the form of reduced service needs or program payments). Subsidies could take the form of tax or direct expenditures proportional to the value placed on the benefits accrued by the public sector.
  —The challenge of ROIs not accruing to specific stakeholders/investors or not accruing fast enough in measuring social services impact and calculating

subsidies, as well as funding and implementing health-related social services, must be addressed.
- Form an entity (similar to MedPAC[13]) that can influence investors to redefine actuarial ROIs, allowing for longer time horizons and a more dedicated focus on collaboration and well-being. This entity would establish common standards and outcome metrics that can be used both for self-accountability and external accountability.
- Create and finance opportunities to improve the health of communities, such as the Healthy Neighborhoods Equity Fund described in Chapter 3 (HNEF, 2022).
- To promote the economic viability of investments that promote whole person health, encourage reporting of financial measures (such as revenue growth) and health measures (such as improved patient-reported outcome measures) over longer time horizons. By de-emphasizing monthly, quarterly, or annual growth, innovative financing models could be given a chance to be fully implemented and delivered before the need for financial returns are required.
- Apply, where possible, an HIA to assess the value of health to financial sector organizations, the impact of specific government or private sector actions on health, and the impact of health or morbidity on a local, community, business, or national level. This assessment may also adopt a framework that accounts for relationships between:
  —An organization's actions and its impact on population health;
  —Population health and its impact on an organization's reputation; and
  —Population health status and its impact on society at large.

Intermediate and Incremental Actions

- Recognize and account for the "wrong pocket problem" in calculations investors make, as payers may not be the sole beneficiaries of the returns accrued.

The following table provides an overview of the Steering Group's judgment of the impact and feasibility of the priority actions described above.

---

[13] The Medicare Payment Advisory Commission (MedPAC) is an "independent congressional agency established by the Balanced Budget Act of 1997 (P.L. 105-33) to advise the U.S. Congress on issues affecting the Medicare program." See https://www.medpac.gov/what-we-do (accessed October 7, 2022).

Priority Action	Category	Impact Rating (1 to 5) 1-least impactful; 5-most impactful	Feasibility Rating (1 to 5) 1-least feasible; 5-most feasible
Create industry and professional standards (e.g., for hospitals, health plan actuaries, and chief financial officers at all health care organizations) that redefine ROI in a way that explicitly quantifies the economic value of health in the population being served.	Transformative	4.0	2.4
In tandem with the right regulatory incentives, partner with a diverse array of entities that benefit from health-related social services to finance them.	Transformative	3.6	2.8
Form an entity (similar to MedPAC) that can influence investors to redefine actuarial ROIs, allowing for longer time horizons and a more dedicated focus on collaboration and well-being.	Transformative	3.6	3.0
Create and finance opportunities to improve the health of communities, such as the HNEF.	Transformative	3.8	3.4
To promote the economic viability of investments that promote whole person health, encourage reporting of financial measures such as revenue growth and health measures such as improved patient-reported outcome measures over longer time horizons.	Transformative	4.4	2.8
Apply, where possible, an HIA that would assess the value of health to financial sector organizations, the impact of specific government or private sector actions on health, and the impact of health or morbidity on a local, community, business, or national level.	Transformative	3.8	2.8
Recognize and account for the "wrong pocket problem" in calculations investors make, as payers may not be the sole beneficiaries of the returns accrued.	Intermediate and Incremental	3	3

CONCLUSION

The path toward creating a nation that values whole person and whole population health in an equitable manner requires more than the sum of the transformative and intermediate/incremental actions described in this chapter. Ultimately, change of this magnitude will require shifts in key principles. First, our system must redefine what it means for individuals, communities, and private enterprises to be successful in today's society. Our current definition of success—quarterly growth, return on investment, and economic gains—must be redefined to, at least in part, recognize the societal value of individual and collective health. Second, each and every stakeholder must leverage their capabilities, invest their resources, and realign incentive structures to promote and purchase health. For example, employers can create conditions to help employees thrive, while clinicians can engage consumers more meaningfully in both personal health and strategy decisions to deliver more meaningful outcomes at the community level. Third, each stakeholder must re-examine the notion of being one entity, organization, or stakeholder whose actions are contained to their specific segment of the system and accept responsibility for their contribution to declining American health and well-being. This realization would open doors for system stakeholders—from insurers and the federal government to the financial sector and patients, families, and communities—to partner and unlock their shared power, volition, and resources to realize the vision of whole person, whole population health. As emphasized by the next chapter, time is of the essence. The nation's continuing health crisis requires transformative, disruptive action to ensure we can stop the backsliding in overall life expectancy, health equity, and health system performance.

REFERENCES

ASTHO (Association of State and Territorial Health Officials). 2022. *Impacting Social Determinants of Health Through Managed Care Contracts.* Available at: https://www.astho.org/topic/population-health-prevention/healthcare-access/medicaid/impacting-sdoh-through-managed-care-contracts (accessed March 2, 2023).

Avanceña, A. L. V., E. K. DeLuca, B. Iott, A. Mauri, N. Miller, D. Eisenberg, and D. W. Dutton. 2021. Income and income inequality are a matter of life and death: What can policymakers do about it? *American Journal of Public Health* 111:1404-1408. https://doi.org/10.2105/AJPH.2021.306301.

Bau, I., R. A. Logan, C. Dezii, B. Rosof, A. Fernandez, M. K. Paasche-Orlow, and W. F. Wong. 2019. Patient-centered, integrated health care quality measures could improve health literacy, language access, and cultural competence. *NAM Perspectives*. Discussion Paper, National Academy of Medicine, Washington, DC. https://doi.org/10.31478/201902a.

Bauchner, H., and P. B. Fontanarosa. 2019. Waste in the US health care system. *JAMA* 322(15):1463-1464. https://doi.org/10.1001/jama.2019.15353. Erratum in *JAMA* 2020 323(6):573. PMID: 31589277.

Berwick, D. M., and A. D. Hackbarth. 2012. Eliminating waste in US health care. *JAMA*. 307(14):1513-1516. https://doi.org/10.1001/jama.2012.362. Epub 2012 Mar 14.

BLS (U.S. Bureau of Labor Statistics). 2022. *The Employment Situation—September 2022*. Available at: https://www.bls.gov/news.release/pdf/empsit.pdf (accessed October 31, 2022).

Bradley, E. H., M. Canavan, E. Roga, K. Talbert-Slagle, C. Ndumele, L. Taylor, and L. A. Curry. 2016. Variation in health outcomes: The role of spending on social services, public health, and health care, 2000-09. *Health Affairs* 35(5):760-768.

Bradley, E. H., H. Sipsma, and L. A. Taylor. 2017. American health care paradox—High spending on health care and poor health, *QJM: An International Journal of Medicine* 110(2):61-65. https://doi.org/10.1093/qjmed/hcw187.

Brookings Health System. 2022. *The Role of Payers*. Available at: https://www.brookingshealth.org/why-brookings-health/health-care-value/understanding-medical-prices/role-payers (accessed October 31, 2022).

Burstin, H., K. Cobb, and K. McQueston. 2017. Measuring what matters to patients: Innovations in integrating the patient experience into development of meaningful performance measures. *National Quality Forum*, August 28.

CAP (Center for American Progress). 2022. *Policies to Hold Nonprofit Hospitals Accountable*. Available at: https://www.americanprogress.org/article/policies-to-hold-nonprofit-hospitals-accountable (accessed March 14, 2023).

Cole, B. L., and J. E. Fielding. 2007. Health impact assessment: A tool to help policy makers understand health beyond health care. *Annual Review of Public Health* 28:393-412. https://doi.org/10.1146/annurev.publhealth.28.083006.131942.

Crook, H. L., R. S. Saunders, R. Roiland, A. Higgins, and M. B. McClellan. 2021. A decade of value-based payment: Lessons learned and implications for the Center for Medicare and Medicaid Innovation, part 2. *Health Affairs Blog*, June 10. https://doi.org/10.1377/forefront.20210607.230763.

Erdelack, L. 2020. Politics, power, and equity. *Health Affairs* 39(6):1095-1096.

Fried, L. P. 2016. Investing in health to create a third demographic dividend. *The Gerontologist* 56(Suppl_2):S167-S177. https://doi.org/10.1093/geront/gnw035.

Gondi, S., and D. A. Chokshi. 2020. Financial stability as a goal of payment reform—a lesson from COVID-19. *JAMA Health Forum* 1(8):e201012.

Held, L. 2022. *Medicaid Is a New Tool to Expand Healthy Food Access*. Available at: https://chlpi.org/news-and-events/news-and-commentary/health-law-and-policy/medicaid-is-a-new-tool-to-expand-healthy-food-access (accessed April 26, 2023).

HNEF (Healthy Neighborhood Equity Fund). 2022. *Investment*. Available at: https://www.hnefund.org/investment (accessed July 28, 2022)

Hyman, D. A., and G. Bai. 2022. *Nonprofit Hospitals' Community Benefits Should Square with Their Tax Exemptions. They Often Don't*. Available at: https://www.cato.org/commentary/nonprofit-hospitals-community-benefits-should-square-their-tax-exemptions-they-often (accessed March 1, 2023).

IOM (Institute of Medicine). 2010. *The Healthcare Imperative: Lowering Costs and Improving Outcomes: Workshop Series Summary*. Washington, DC: The National Academies Press. https://doi.org/10.17226/12750.

IOM. 2015. *Vital Signs: Core Metrics for Health and Health Care Progress*. Washington, DC: The National Academies Press. https://doi.org/10.17226/19402.

Lallemand, N. C. 2012. Reducing waste in health care. *Health Affairs Blog*, December 13. https://doi.org/10.1377/hpb20121213.959735.

Levy, J. F., B. N. Ippolito, and A. Jain. Hospital revenue under Maryland's total cost of care model during the COVID-19 pandemic, March-July 2020. *JAMA* 325(4):398-400. https://doi.org/10.1001/jama.2020.22149.

Liaw, W., A. W. Bazemore, and R. L. Phillips. 2017. Aggregation to promote health in an era of data and value based payment healthcare. 5(3):92-94. https://doi.org/10.1016/j.hjdsi.2017.05.004.

Majerol, M., and D. L. Hughes. 2022. *CMS Innovation Center Tackles Implicit Bias*. Available at: https://www.healthaffairs.org/do/10.1377/forefront.20220630.238592 (accessed March 1, 2023).

MPHA (Massachusetts Public Health Association). 2019. *Prevention and Wellness Trust Fund*. Available at: https://mapublichealth.org/priorities/pwtf (accessed March 14, 2023).

MSCI. 2022. *The Global Industry Classification Standard (GICS®)*. Available at: https://www.msci.com/our-solutions/indexes/gics (accessed October 31, 2022).

NASEM (National Academies of Sciences, Engineering, and Medicine). 2016. *Systems Practices for the Care of Socially At-Risk Populations*. Washington, DC: The National Academies Press. https://doi.org/10.17226/21914.

NASEM. 2019. *Integrating Social Care into the Delivery of Health Care: Moving Upstream to Improve the Nation's Health*. Washington, DC: The National Academies Press. https://doi.org/10.17226/25467.

NASEM. 2021a. *Implementing High-Quality Primary Care: Rebuilding the Foundation of Health Care.* Washington, DC: The National Academies Press. https://doi.org/10.17226/25983.

NASEM. 2021b. *Financing That Rewards Better Health and Well-Being: Proceedings of a Workshop—in Brief.* Washington, DC: The National Academies Press. https://doi.org/10.17226/26332.

NOLA Coalition. 2022. *The Mission.* https://nolacoalition.info (accessed July 20, 2022).

One Percent Steps for Health Care Reform. 2022. *Policy Briefs.* https://onepercentsteps.com/policy-briefs (accessed June 21, 2022).

Oregon Health Authority. 2023. *In Lieu of Services.* Available at: https://www.oregon.gov/oha/HSD/OHP/Pages/ILOS.aspx (accessed March 2, 2023).

Podulka, J., and Y. Narayan. 2021. *Center for Medicare and Medicaid Innovation: Findings from Medicare Models to-Date.* Available at: https://www.healthmanagement.com/wp-content/uploads/HMA-AV-Issue-Brief-1-CMMI-findings.pdf (accessed October 13, 2022).

Rubin, J., J. Taylor, J. Krapels, A. Sutherland, M. Felician, J. Liu, L. Davis, and C. Rohr. 2016. *Are Better Health Outcomes Related to Social Expenditure? A Cross-National Empirical Analysis of Social Expenditure and Population Health Measures.* Santa Monica, CA: RAND Corporation, 2016. Available at: https://www.rand.org/pubs/research_reports/RR1252.html (accessed September 1, 2022).

Sharfstein, J. M., S. Gerovich, E. Moriarty, and D. Chin. 2017. An emerging approach to payment reform: All-payer global budgets for large safety-net hospital systems. *The Commonwealth Fund,* August. https://doi.org/10.26099/95nm-hj53.

Shrank, W. H., T. L. Rogstad, and N. Parekh. 2019. Waste in the US health care system: Estimated costs and potential for savings. *JAMA* 322(15):1501-1509. https://doi.org/10.1001/jama.2019.13978.

Shrank, W. H., N. A. DeParle, S. Gottlieb, S. H. Jain, P. Orszag, B. W. Powers, and G. R. Wilensky. 2021. Health costs and financing: Challenges and strategies for a new administration: Commentary recommends health cost, financing, and other priorities for a new US administration. *Health Affairs* 40(2):235-242.

Siblis Research. 2022. *Total Market Value of the U.S. Stock Market.* Available at: https://siblisresearch.com/data/us-stock-market-value (accessed October 31, 2022).

Smith, B. 2021. CMS Innovation Center at 10 years—progress and lessons learned. *New England Journal of Medicine* 384(8):759-764. https://doi.org/10.1056/NEJMsb2031138. Epub 2021 Jan 13.

The White House. 2022a. *The Legislative Branch.* Available at: https://www.whitehouse.gov/about-the-white-house/our-government/the-legislative-branch (accessed November 1, 2022).

The White House. 2022b. *The Executive Branch*. Available at: https://www.whitehouse.gov/about-the-white-house/our-government/the-executive-branch (accessed November 1, 2022).

Urban Institute. 2021. *State and Local Backgrounders*. Available at: https://www.urban.org/policy-centers/cross-center-initiatives/state-and-local-finance-initiative/state-and-local-backgrounders/state-and-local-expenditures (accessed October 31, 2022).

Urban Institute. 2022. *Blended and Braided Funding*. Available at: https://wfguide.urban.org/node/57.html (accessed March 2, 2023).

5

HEALTH TRANSFORMATION THROUGH DISRUPTIVE CHANGE

American health is declining and its health system is fractured. Accelerated by the COVID-19 pandemic but also due to pervasive issues such as systemic racism, structural wealth inequality and poverty, deaths of despair, and the U.S.' crumbling-to-nonexistent social infrastructure, our health will likely continue to decline without fundamental, some would say radical, change. Though evidence and models of what works to improve health exist, society continues to invest resources and attention in approaches that do not significantly improve health and well-being.

To reverse this concerning trend, health and health care leaders, as well as other stakeholders, must recognize that the incremental steps of the past several decades have not led to significant progress. The public health system continues to be underfunded, understaffed, and fragmented. The health care system continues to grow in size and financial magnitude, but despite ever-increasing resources, it does not seem capable of making investments to improve population health. This is largely because the health care system is stuck in the status quo—an ingrained "medical care" mindset exacerbated by misaligned incentives. As it stands today, the system lacks sufficient leadership and alignment to move in a different direction without additional action.

The time for incrementalism is over. Americans must act quickly and collectively to appropriately value our health and change how we conceive of health and well-being going forward and shape the conditions that promote it. The urgency that has propelled change in responding to the climate crisis must now fuel how health and health care leaders consider our nation's health.

We do not have much time. Disruptive change is needed in who, what, and how we finance, pay for, and ultimately value health. If the slow, incremental pace of change continues, we cannot expect significant progress toward greater equity, improved life span, or quality of life. Instead, we will continue to spend more on care that only marginally impacts health while neglecting other areas with an outsized influence on our collective well-being.

However, this does not have to be our future. While the comparatively dire state of our nation's health is due to fragmented incentives, values, and systems prioritizing the bottom line over health, the solution lies in uniting our communities, governance structures, and businesses. This movement begins with patients, families, and communities demanding that policy makers take bold, disruptive steps to prioritize individual and collective health in all policies. As all sectors implement policies, incentives, and regulations that support a system-wide transformation toward whole person, whole population health as described in Chapter 4, they will direct action and alignment toward a rapid and voluminous creation of solutions.

The transformation spurred by these incentives and policies should manifest through large volumes of new public and private capital to invest in health-producing solutions. In Chapter 4, the Steering Group proposed a set of goals to strive for by 2030, along with opportunities for action that key stakeholders can take to reverse the current trajectory and begin a movement toward whole health in the United States. By implementing these priority actions, the right incentives and the necessary conditions would be created to prompt every sector to change how they do business. Most importantly, these solutions would center health at the forefront of every decision and policy. In every sector, leaders should set ambitious health-related goals and be held accountable for striving to meet them.

While this transformation in health may sound radical or implausible, we are witnessing an example on this scale through activism on climate change. Although more progress needs to be made, the case for climate action is approaching wide acceptance as new policy and cultural norms have been established. Today, leadership is rising from sectors including retail, transportation, financing, architecture and building construction, and farming. These partnerships and actions have emerged in different forms as more organizations realize they have important roles in mitigating climate change. The same type of broad-based activism and change leadership is needed for our nation's health. Appendix C describes a possible cascade of change starting with action from the federal government.

An activated citizenry is the key to change. Without a mass social movement that pushes leaders, organizations, and sectors at each and every level to prioritize health in every policy; radically transforms the involvement of every stakeholder in health promotion and prevention; and promotes financing and paying for health care that promotes whole health, the authors believe that the national health crisis will continue to fester. The present approach will be the same incremental steps we have seen, which have not succeeded in substantially mitigating health disparities or stopping the decline in national health.

A multi-stakeholder approach is also needed for significant change to occur. While the federal and state governments must set bold goals and align policies and incentives with whole health, action from other organizations such as social service and anchor institutions, as well as care delivery organizations and payers, is necessary to realize the vision of this Special Publication. This transformation will only happen when the government is pushed by its citizenry to act and lead boldly.

As the conditions for change emerge, the best and boldest solutions may not come from the health care and public health sectors. Because there is little incentive for health care leaders to change the status quo, it is highly unlikely that the industry alone will lead the needed changes. Leadership will likely come from community leaders, philanthropy, business leaders, investors, and change-makers within the health care industry who see the value of investing in health. Regardless, the conditions must exist for *all* entities to be incentivized to invest in and advance whole person and population health. As communities begin to experience the benefit of better health, the authors hope that a positive feedback cycle will result in more entities prioritizing health and doing business in new and different ways that lead to better overall health.

Investors can see the return on investment (ROI) of financing changes that lead to healthier communities and healthy returns. Private equity and venture capital are now pouring billions of dollars into health care companies—in 2018, the valuation of private equity deals for the health care sector surpassed $100 billion (Offodile et al., 2021). Investments in health care continue to be attractive precisely because the incentives for realizing a system of *health care* are currently so enticing. Health care is recession-resistant, many operational and outcomes gaps require potentially profitable and innovative solutions, and an aging population could lead to higher care utilization (Offodile et al., 2021). While the impact of novel technologies or care models on overall health is still largely unknown, the rapid and deep investment signals that the private sector will continue to value these investments when financial incentives and potential ROI are aligned. Many of the priority actions outlined in this publication are intended to do just that: align incentives with *health* rather than health care for its own sake and establish the utility of measuring ROI based on overall long-term improvement in whole person and whole population health.

Collective action, though difficult, has the potential to produce meaningful and disruptive change that will improve American health. Working together to fix this national health crisis holds enormous potential for cost savings, capital gains, and real economic growth. If the climate crisis is worth changing how we do business for the sake of future generations, so is creating the conditions for everyone and every community to experience their most healthy state. The way is clear; what is needed now is the will to move forward.

REFERENCE

Offodile, A. C. II, M. Cerullo, M. Bindal, J. A. Rauh-Hainn, and V. Ho. 2021. Private equity investments in health care: An overview of hospital and health system leveraged buyouts, 2003-17. *Health Affairs* 40(5):719-726.

Appendix A

FINANCING THAT REWARDS BETTER HEALTH AND WELL-BEING WORKSHOP SERIES PARTICIPANT SUGGESTIONS

In the spring of 2021, under the auspices of the National Academy of Medicine's (NAM's) Leadership Consortium in collaboration with the National Academies of Sciences, Engineering, and Medicine's (the National Academies') Health and Medicine Division, a 3-day workshop series titled Financing That Rewards Better Health and Well-Being was held (NASEM, 2021). A Proceedings of a Workshop—in Brief (PIB), which highlighted presentations and discussions from the workshop, was published in September 2021 (NASEM, 2021). Important themes from the workshop, as interpreted by authors of this publication, as well as proposed implementation actions from the PIB are briefly summarized below.

WORKSHOP THEMES

1. The current system of paying for health care is not designed to reward improved health outcomes and is especially inadequate in advancing the health of vulnerable populations with low incomes.
2. Policies and strategies that encompass both clinical and nonclinical approaches that can promote optimal health and well-being exist, but they are limited in scope and scale, which limits their growth and sustainability in the current payment system.
3. New funding and finance strategies are needed to disrupt dysfunctional health care delivery pathways and support approaches that work to improve health.
4. Effective approaches to improving health will necessitate more than innovative care models and sometimes lie entirely outside the health and health care sectors.

Reimagining Approaches to Care for the Entire Population

- Integrate services that drive health and well-being.
- Extend domains of care to encompass communities.
- Invest in health care and social supports for infants and children to address health disparities that occur early in life.
- Engage in effective life-stage care strategies.
- Provide high-quality care to older adults and individuals with disabilities.
- Expand the use of home- and community-based services.
- Make full use of telehealth, virtual health, and other technologies.

Redesigning Health Financing to Focus on Producing Whole Person and Whole Population Health and Well-Being

- Establish health system accountability based on meaningful quality measures.
- Invest in a workforce that can provide whole person and whole population health.
- Leverage state, local, and federal funding opportunities to experiment, authorize, assess, and extend care delivery and financing innovations.
- Set longer time horizons for returns on investments in health.
- Use universal empanelment[1] to provide high-quality primary care.
- Use lessons from the COVID-19 pandemic to recognize gaps and the fragility of fee-for-service financing strategies, and transition away from their use.
- Connect the public- and private-sector producers of better health with the entities interested in investing in better health to direct resources to address the social determinants of health.
- Shift resources toward vulnerable populations with low incomes to improve population health and lower the costs of health care.
- Leverage market forces to aid the health system in moving away from fee-for-service financing structures.
- Implement mandatory payment strategies that do not operate on fee-for-service business models.
- Eliminate frictional costs[2] and "gaming the system."

---

[1] Empanelment refers to a "continuous, iterative set of processes that identify and assign populations to practices, care teams, or clinicians that have a responsibility to know their assigned population and proactively deliver coordinated primary care" (Bearden et al., 2019; NASEM, 2021, p. 312).

[2] Frictional costs refer to the total financial transaction costs—both direct and indirect—incurred beyond the actual cost of the service or product.

Cross-Cutting Suggestions

- Ensure that equity is a major driver of transformed health care delivery and financing.
- Study how relationships in complex systems give rise to collective behaviors to learn how to redirect those systems.
- Create a shared digital infrastructure to enable better communication, coordination, data sharing, and strategic investments.
- Build on collaborative, cross-sector partnerships to advance better health and well-being.
- Ensure that patients are at the center of payment and care.

REFERENCES

Bearden, T., H. L. Ratcliffe, J. R. Sugarman, A. Bitton, L. A. Anaman, G. Buckle, M. Cham, D. Chong Woei Quan, F. Ismail, B. Jargalsaikhan, W. Lim, N. M. Mohammad, I. C. N. Morrison, B. Norov, J. Oh, G. Riimaadai, S. Sararaks, and L. R. Hirschhorn. 2019. Empanelment: A foundational component of primary health care. *Gates Open Research* 3:1654. https://doi.org/10.12688/gatesopenres.13059.1

NASEM (National Academies of Sciences, Engineering, and Medicine). 2021a. *Financing That Rewards Better Health and Well-Being: Proceedings of a Workshop—in Brief.* Washington, DC: The National Academies Press. https://doi.org/10.17226/26332.

Appendix B

STAKEHOLDER-SPECIFIC PRIORITY ACTIONS BY IMPACT AND FEASIBILITY

The following tables provide an overview of the Steering Group's judgment of the impact and feasibility of the stakeholder-specific priority actions outlined in Chapter 4.[1]

PATIENTS, FAMILIES, AND COMMUNITIES

Priority Action	Category	Impact Rating (1 to 5) 1–least impactful; 5–most impactful	Feasibility Rating (1 to 5) 1–least feasible; 5–most feasible
Harness the political process and advocate for financial reforms and more equitable and inclusive health policies.	Transformative	4.4	2.6
Engage in advocacy skills training to enhance the power of the whole person, whole population health movement by expanding stakeholder networks.	Intermediate and Incremental	2.8	3.6
Develop and participate in community-based, multi-stakeholder coalitions to guide the design, implementation, and evaluation of programs to support whole person and whole population health and well-being.	Intermediate and Incremental	3.2	3.4

---

[1] See the publication's Acronyms and Abbreviations section for an explanation of acronyms used throughout Appendix B.

Ensure that a diverse array of community members is involved in the governance of local, state, and/or regional health coalitions to improve equity, inclusion, and representation as it pertains to race, ethnicity, age, and disability status, among other personal characteristics.	Intermediate and Incremental	3.0	3.2
Educate stakeholders on the need to advocate for policies that prioritize whole health, including the indirect impacts of other policy decisions on health.	Intermediate and Incremental	2.8	3.6

State and Local Governments

Legislative and Executive Branches

Priority Action	Category	Impact Rating (1 to 5) 1-least impactful; 5-most impactful	Feasibility Rating (1 to 5) 1-least feasible; 5-most feasible
Pursue and use 1115 waivers to cover innovative care and payment models that address social determinants of health.	Transformative	3.6	4.0
Require managed care organizations to focus on prevention and social determinants of health through Medicaid managed care contracts.	Transformative	3.4	4.0
Use accountable care organization models to assign providers responsibility for the costs and quality of a defined community's health.	Transformative	3.4	3.0
Align policies across state health insurance programs like Medicaid, Children's Health Insurance Program, and state employee insurance, as well as between state insurance programs and state social service entities to better support health outcomes.	Transformative	3.4	2.8

Require that all nonprofit hospitals engage in multi-stakeholder collaborations to establish and finance locally controlled pools of funds with a neutral community entity as a fiscal agent similar to the Massachusetts Prevention & Wellness Trust Fund program.	Transformative	4.6	3.2
Design and require the use of HIAs to assess the impact of policy proposals and business activities on health, particularly in sectors where health impacts may not be currently considered.	Transformative	3.4	3.4
Develop, or require the development of, cross-sector, data-sharing capabilities to facilitate cross-platform collaboration between public health, insurance, social services, and care delivery information systems.	Transformative	3.4	2.6
Require nonprofit health systems to apply community benefit dollars toward impact investments that improve social, economic, and environmental conditions in disadvantaged communities while also producing economic returns for investors.	Intermediate and Incremental	3.3	3.8

Community Benefit Oversight

Priority Action	Category	Impact Rating (1 to 5) 1-least impactful; 5-most impactful	Feasibility Rating (1 to 5) 1-least feasible; 5-most feasible
Set performance goals to improve health outcomes and transform nonprofit hospitals' approaches to consumer engagement and care.	Transformative	3.8	3.0
Amplify baseline federal requirements to promote meaningful engagement of cross-sector and/or community-governed collaborations as key components in CHNAs and CHAs.	Intermediate and Incremental	2.6	3.2

Priority Action	Category	Impact	Feasibility
Require the standardization and integration of CHNAs conducted by hospitals within the same health system to yield robust data on unmet health and health-related social needs within a designated service area.	Intermediate and Incremental	2.4	3.8
Leverage state authority to make appointments to the boards of public hospitals that ensure meaningful community representation.	Intermediate and Incremental	2.0	3.8
Use certificate of need decisions to address inequities and disparities relating to access to primary care, geographic location, race, ethnicity, disability status, etc.	Intermediate and Incremental	3.0	3.2

Insurance Oversight

Priority Action	Category	Impact Rating (1 to 5) *1-least impactful; 5-most impactful*	Feasibility Rating (1 to 5) *1-least feasible; 5-most feasible*
Adopt and expand laws and regulations pertaining to health insurance rate review and, specifically, approval authority.	Transformative	4.2	3.2
Leverage state insurance department approval processes to institute usual source of care requirements for fully insured health plans.	Intermediate and Incremental	3.0	3.3

Appropriations

Priority Action	Category	Impact Rating (1 to 5) *1-least impactful; 5-most impactful*	Feasibility Rating (1 to 5) *1-least feasible; 5-most feasible*
Place unspent government funds from pandemic-era legislation such as the American Rescue Plan Act into community-governed pools and allow service beneficiaries and navigators to govern their use toward upstream determinants of health and social services.	Transformative	3.6	2.8
Earmark funds for structured training at the local level to strengthen political and health literacy, as well as civic engagement and community governance skills.	Intermediate and Incremental	2.8	3.4

Public Health Agencies and Departments

Priority Action	Category	Impact Rating (1 to 5) *1-least impactful; 5-most impactful*	Feasibility Rating (1 to 5) *1-least feasible; 5-most feasible*
Lead the development of community-wide goals and collective impact strategies to improve health and equity, involving multiple government agencies, nonprofit partners, and the private sector. Support the full engagement of community residents in the process.	Transformative	4.0	2.4
Partner with health care organizations incentivized to better health outcomes to codevelop and lead community programs that advance prevention. Support the full engagement of community residents and local organizations in the process.	Transformative	4.0	3.8

Lead coordination of CHAs and CHNAs, so that they provide opportunities for meaningful engagement of community residents, address key determinants of health, and advance prevention across the community, shifting collective emphasis away from individual conditions (such as diabetes and heart disease) to community infrastructure that better supports health.	Intermediate and Incremental	3.2	3.4
Create protocols for systematically assessing the capacity of community health and social service providers to determine how the community as a whole can address service gaps in an efficient, collective, and sustainable way.	Intermediate and Incremental	2.4	3.6
Utilize public health authority as appropriate to allow community-supported strategies to have the greatest impact.	Intermediate and Incremental	2.5	2.3

Federal Government

Priority Action	Category	Impact Rating (1 to 5) 1-least impactful; 5-most impactful	Feasibility Rating (1 to 5) 1-least feasible; 5-most feasible
Expand ACA requirements governing "essential benefits" for plans sold in the individual and small group markets.	Transformative	4.2	2.8
Review ERISA and large group insurance requirements to add integrative care and home and community services and supports as essential benefits.	Transformative	3.6	2.6
Revise the medical loss ratios used in the ACA to become "health loss ratios" that support health rather than health care.	Transformative	4.4	3.0
Design and require the use of health impact assessments to assess the impact of policy proposals and business activities on health, particularly in sectors where health impacts may not be currently considered.	Transformative	3.8	2.8

Supplement federal health care reform efforts to create a federal benefits package that incentivizes an expanded or reconsidered set of "essential benefits."	Transformative	4.0	2.8
Require that all nonprofit hospitals engage in multi-stakeholder collaborations to establish and finance locally controlled pools of funds with a neutral community entity as a fiscal agent.	Transformative	3.8	2.4
Require nonprofit health systems to apply community benefit dollars toward impact investments that improve social, economic, and environmental conditions in disadvantaged communities.	Transformative	3.4	3.4
Create a parsimonious set of quality measures that provide meaningful information on person-centered health and well-being outcomes.	Transformative	3.6	4.4
Require a 2% to 5% withholding from current federal grants to state programs to create a flexible federally funded pool for which localities or states could apply to implement community-governed whole person health improvement strategies.	Transformative	3.6	3.2
CMS should stop paying for interventions or services not proven to improve health outcomes and increase scrutiny of new and existing therapeutics, adjusting their reimbursement policies accordingly.	Transformative	3.4	3.2
Create a funding pool modeled off the CMMI State Innovation Model that would incentivize less-resourced states or regions to adopt population-based global budgets, specifically focusing on improving children's health, as communities, health care payers, and providers often need financial support to transition to innovative payment models that support whole person care (e.g., all-payer global budgets).	Intermediate and Incremental	2.8	3.4
Increase funding and support for programs that address health-related social factors.	Intermediate and Incremental	3.0	2.6
Create a commission to deliver recommendations to Congress on how to restructure existing health and social service programs to bring greater value to consumers and taxpayers.	Intermediate and Incremental	2.0	4.4

Priority Action	Category	Impact	Feasibility
Strengthen and optimize CHNAs to center on community-governed interventions and funding in order to enhance collective financing mechanisms listed in the previous section.	Intermediate and Incremental	3.2	3.8
Pioneer the development and implementation of payment models based on priorities of CBOs and designed with their partnership.	Intermediate and Incremental	3.2	3.2

Care Delivery Organizations and Health Systems

Priority Action	Category	Impact Rating (1 to 5) *1-least impactful; 5-most impactful*	Feasibility Rating (1 to 5) *1-least feasible; 5-most feasible*
Transform the landscape of economic incentives to support whole person health by transitioning 75% of the health system reimbursement framework to population-based payments.	Transformative	4.6	2.2
Pursue multilevel approaches to working collaboratively with community stakeholders, such as fair compensation for community health workers, credibly and meaningfully integrating community voices into health system strategy and decision-making, and building meaningful alliances with a broad ecosystem of community organizations.	Transformative	3.8	2.6
Invest in information technology infrastructure that can catalyze gains in community health, such as robust information exchange and data-sharing processes between care delivery organizations and CBOs, as well as "digital front doors" (i.e., health kiosks) in the community.	Transformative	3.4	3.4
Screen patients for social determinants of health and health-related social needs and provide closed-loop referrals to social service entities and CBOs that can meet those needs.	Transformative	4.2	4.5

Set goals for an increased amount of community benefit dollars and grants spent on evidence-based services and strategies that strengthen whole person, whole population health and well-being.	Intermediate and Incremental	3.2	3.6
Align the compensation structure of senior executives to health system performance on a set of community defined health metrics.	Intermediate and Incremental	3.2	2.2
Establish a community liaison infrastructure within the health system to align activities and create shared expectations with CBOs.	Intermediate and Incremental	2.8	3.4

Payers

Priority Action	Category	Impact Rating (1 to 5) 1-least impactful; 5-most impactful	Feasibility Rating (1 to 5) 1-least feasible; 5-most feasible
Establish processes to routinely identify the social needs of the health plan members and direct investments toward resources to address those needs.	Transformative	4.3	4.4
Create a population health business model where private payers such as commercial health insurance plans, insurance plan providers, health systems, and, if possible, CMS pay CBOs to create value and improve health and well-being by facilitating healthy opportunities.	Transformative	4.4	3.4
Evaluate and expand on the scope of "essential benefits" required under the ACA to include guaranteed coverage for services that produce whole health and well-being.	Transformative	3.8	3.2
Reimburse care delivery organizations, social service entities, and community-based organizations for closed-loop referrals targeting member social determinants of health and health-related social needs.	Transformative	3.4	3.2
Hold health systems accountable to anchor organization practices that will promote whole person, whole population health through payer-provider contracts.	Transformative	3.8	2.0

Priority Action	Category	Impact	Feasibility
Pioneer the development and implementation of payment models based on priorities of CBOs and designed with their partnership.	Intermediate and Incremental	3.2	3.2
Build alliances with key community partners (e.g., law enforcement, emergency response, criminal justice, schools, and social services providers) that encourage cooperation within the local ecosystem to support outcomes aligned with the Quintuple Aim.	Intermediate and Incremental	3.2	4.0
Reduce practice consolidation by implementing payment policies inclusive of small, independent health care practices.	Intermediate and Incremental	2.8	4.0

Employers

Priority Action	Category	Impact Rating (1 to 5) 1–least impactful; 5–most impactful	Feasibility Rating (1 to 5) 1–least feasible; 5–most feasible
Enhance workforce well-being by establishing an expanded set of "essential benefits" in health benefit packages provided to employees that includes relevant social services.	Transformative	4.0	3.8
Establish linkages and partnerships with health care, local government, CBOs, and philanthropies that leverage employers' position as community cornerstones, which includes: their ability to influence individual employees within and outside the workplace; their power as purchasers of health plans; and the impact of their businesses on the local environment.	Transformative	3.4	3.6
Join forces to apply employers' collective economic power in their communities to address health-related social challenges impacting members of the community, including employees.	Transformative	3.4	3.0
Capitalize on sector market power to purchase health plans that provide access to closed-loop referrals that target members' health-related social needs.	Intermediate and Incremental	3.3	3.5

Set minimum expectations for how health plans should contract and collaborate with CBOs.	Intermediate and Incremental	2.6	2.6
Incentivize employees through employer-purchased health plans to seek care from in-network practitioners with expertise in health behavior change, healthy lifestyles, and wellness (e.g., lifestyle medicine, integrative medicine).	Intermediate and Incremental	2.8	2.6

Financial Sector Organizations

Priority Action	Category	Impact Rating (1 to 5) 1-least impactful; 5-most impactful	Feasibility Rating (1 to 5) 1-least feasible; 5-most feasible
Create industry and professional standards (e.g., for hospitals, health plan actuaries, and chief financial officers at all health care organizations) that redefine ROI in a way that explicitly quantifies the economic value of health in the population being served.	Transformative	4.0	2.4
In tandem with the right regulatory incentives, partner with a diverse array of entities that benefit from health-related social services to finance them.	Transformative	3.6	2.8
Form an entity (similar to MedPAC) that can influence investors to redefine actuarial ROIs, allowing for longer time horizons and a more dedicated focus on collaboration and well-being.	Transformative	3.6	3.0
Create and finance opportunities to improve the health of communities, such as the HNEF.	Transformative	3.8	3.4
To promote the economic viability of investments that promote whole person health, encourage reporting of financial measures such as revenue growth and health measures such as improved patient-reported outcome measures over longer time horizons.	Transformative	4.4	2.8

Apply, where possible, an HIA that would assess the value of health to financial sector organizations, the impact of specific government or private sector actions on health, and the impact of health or morbidity on a local, community, business, or national level.	Transformative	3.8	2.8
Recognize and account for the "wrong pocket problem" in calculations investors make, as payers may not be the sole beneficiaries of the returns accrued.	Intermediate and Incremental	3.0	3.0

REFERENCES

Bearden, T., H. L. Ratcliffe, J. R. Sugarman, A. Bitton, L. A. Anaman, G. Buckle, M. Cham, D. Chong Woei Quan, F. Ismail, B. Jargalsaikhan, W. Lim, N. M. Mohammad, I. C. N. Morrison, B. Norov, J. Oh, G. Riimaadai, S. Sararaks, and L. R. Hirschhorn. 2019. Empanelment: A foundational component of primary health care. *Gates Open Research* 3:1654. https://doi.org/10.12688/gatesopenres.13059.1

NASEM (National Academies of Sciences, Engineering, and Medicine). 2021. *Financing That Rewards Better Health and Well-Being: Proceedings of a Workshop—in Brief.* Washington, DC: The National Academies Press. https://doi.org/10.17226/26332.

Appendix C

ILLUSTRATIVE MODELS OF IMPLEMENTING WHOLE PERSON, WHOLE POPULATION HEALTH PRIORITY ACTIONS

This appendix was drafted by the Steering Committee to exemplify how an activated citizenry could begin leveraging the political process, pushing leaders in the federal government to act, and holding them accountable for progress as raised in Chapter 4. Through the examples of ending housing instability and food insecurity, this section outlines how action by the federal government can spur action in other sectors.

DISRUPTIVE ACTION TO ADDRESS HOUSING INSTABILITY

FEDERAL MANDATES AND PRIORITIES

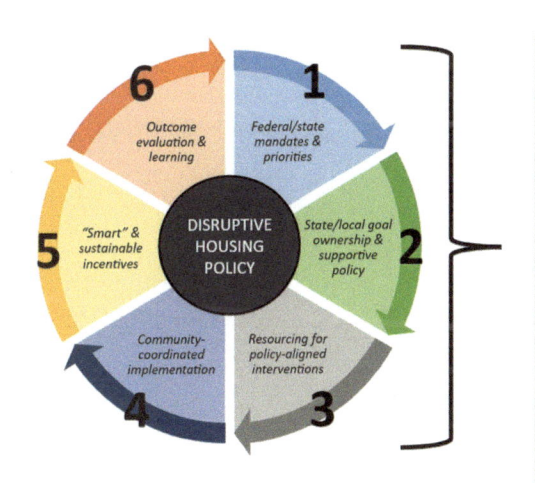

EXAMPLE BENEFITS
- More stable housing for individuals/families
- Reduction of downstream health effects/interacting social needs
- Lower health care spending
- Community-guided real estate and development
- New investment opportunities
- Lower crime rates
- Business opportunities for builders
- Healthier, more stable workforce
- Higher school attendance and success

Wheel diagram of DISRUPTIVE HOUSING POLICY:
1. Federal/state mandates & priorities
2. State/local goal ownership & supportive policy
3. Resourcing for policy-aligned interventions
4. Community-coordinated implementation
5. "Smart" & sustainable incentives
6. Outcome evaluation & learning

FIGURE 5 Sample dynamics of disruptive policy | housing stability.

In response to national advocacy demanding whole person, whole population health interventions, federal government leaders could first set bold goals and corresponding policy changes to drive demand for solutions to these seemingly intractable problems. For example, the federal government could set the following bold national goals related to housing:

- Eliminate childhood homelessness nationally;
- Reduce adult homelessness by 75 percent; and
- Ensure no one must spend more than 30 percent of their income on housing costs.

Existing federal policies would then be changed either legislatively or through regulation to align with these goals. For example, the tax code or Medicare and Medicaid policy could be harnessed to create strong incentives and disincentives that align with these goals (see Box 4).

BOX 4

Housing Stability: Aligning Federal Policies with the Vision for Whole Person, Whole Population Health

- Index federal business tax rates to the rate of homelessness and average percent of income spent on housing costs in a given county or state.
- Adjust Medicare Area Wage Index to reward areas with affordable housing and low homelessness rates. Similarly adjust Medicaid Federal Medical Assistance Percentage (FMAP) calculations.
- Align federal tax rates for top bracket of income earners and real estate purchases of >$1M to homelessness and housing burden for a given state or county.
- Apply tax penalties based on percentage of units in a real estate development that cost more than what the median (or 25th percentile) income earner in the market can afford with 30 percent of their income.
- Further apply tax penalties for home sales of investors while exempting owner.
- Implement tax deductions for favorable actions like development of majority-affordable housing complexes or making personal investments in housing-forward businesses (a new IRS classification).
- Allow health insurers to count housing support as part of their medical loss ratio.

Assessing progress toward initial goals will help to inform federal and state priorities moving forward. Starting points could include the following:

- Monitor chronic homelessness and other forms of housing insecurity with an approach like the U.S. Department of Housing and Urban Development's (HUD's) point-in-time estimates.
- Track housing affordability through well-established survey methods. The Census Bureau could conduct this data collection and analysis every 2-3 years.
- Track waiting times for people eligible for housing assistance.

STATE AND LOCAL GOVERNMENT ALIGNMENT

With incentives and penalties in place at the federal level, state and local government leaders should begin to experience pressure from businesses, Medicare and Medicaid providers, real estate developers, and others to conform to state and local policies that align with federal housing priorities. Local governments may then begin to:

- Change zoning laws to support higher density and more affordable developments;
- Remove regulatory barriers to multifamily housing units; and
- Place caps on growth in land prices.

PUBLIC AND PRIVATE FINANCING OF SOLUTIONS

In response to new financial incentives put in place by the federal government, public and private financing should also begin to shift in support of affordable housing. For example, one might begin to see:

- Real Estate Investment Trusts (REITs) diversify to invest in the development of affordable housing;
- Institutional investors link portfolio decisions to homelessness and housing affordability;
- Venture investors prioritize Medicare Advantage and Medicaid health plans that have housing solutions and companies that build affordable prefabricated homes;
- Local health systems repurpose their underused real estate to lease to low-income patients and others at risk for homelessness;
- New real estate developers specialize in working with community stakeholders and building affordable housing as in-fills or in new areas;

- New partnerships between health systems and real estate developers emerge; and
- Healthy neighborhood equity funds move quickly to identify high-value land and make upstream investments to create more value for existing residents versus new residents.

INVESTMENTS DIRECTED BY EMPOWERED COMMUNITY STAKEHOLDERS

In addition to public and private financing shifting to support more affordable housing, community stakeholders should also drive investment decisions and capital allocation. Governing bodies of key community stakeholders should be established locally to help guide important investment decisions. For example:

- Working with local government planners, community stakeholders could identify geographic areas to prioritize for housing investments and types of housing or development.
- Investors should be able to easily access such maps to make commitments.
- Discounted auctions should be created for community-based trusts to purchase critical real estate and thus make decisions surrounding allocations, scale, use, and development.

SUSTAINABLE SOLUTIONS

To ensure the sustainability of the interventions, thoughtfully designed incentive structures should be created and implemented. These should be flexible enough to reward different outcomes over time and effectively designed so they visibly sustain activities that produce favored outcomes. The solutions should pay for themselves if effective land and development costs, inclusive of claimed tax burdens and deductions, are low enough to generate reasonable profit based on purchases limited to 30 percent of income. It is reasonable to expect that as homelessness and housing instability decrease, overall behavioral health outcomes will improve, even though substantial wraparound behavioral health care services are required nationally.

The same activism around food insecurity could also lead to improved whole health.

DISRUPTIVE ACTION TO ADDRESS FOOD INSECURITY

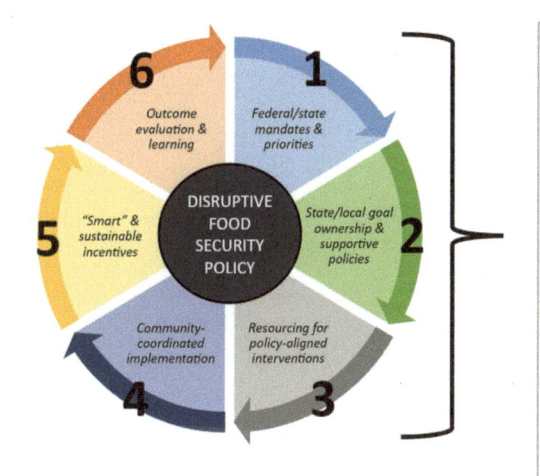

EXAMPLE BENEFITS
- Better nutrition for individuals/families
- Reduction of downstream health effects/interacting social needs
- Lower health care spending
- Markets for locally produced food and employment opportunities
- New investment opportunities
- Lower crime rates
- Business opportunities for vendors of nutritious food
- Healthier, more stable workforce
- Higher school attendance and success

Wheel diagram centered on "DISRUPTIVE FOOD SECURITY POLICY" with six segments:
1. Federal/state mandates & priorities
2. State/local goal ownership & supportive policies
3. Resourcing for policy-aligned interventions
4. Community-coordinated implementation
5. "Smart" & sustainable incentives
6. Outcome evaluation & learning

FIGURE 6 | Sample dynamics of disruptive policy | food security.

FEDERAL MANDATES AND PRIORITIES

To advance whole person, whole population health, leaders in the federal government could begin a transformation in this area by setting the following bold national goals related to food insecurity:

- Eliminate childhood food insecurity;
- Reduce adult individual and household food insecurity by 90 percent; and
- Ensure no household must spend more than 30 percent of its income on food, and all households have access to adequate nutrition to thrive.

Existing federal policies would then be changed either legislatively or through regulation to align with these goals (see Box 5).

BOX 5

Food Security: Aligning Federal Policies with the Vision for Whole Person, Whole Population Health

- Tie business tax rates, at higher levels of income, to the level or improvement in the rate of food insecurity in a given state or county.
- Provide federal income tax breaks on the percentage of income spent on food by low-income households in a given state or county.
- Adjust Medicaid Federally Medical Assistance Percentage (FMAP) to the percentage of income spent on food by low-income households in a given state or county. Provide bonus FMAP if no county within the state has food insecurity greater than 5 percent.
- Tie FMAP bonus to the level of SNAP eligibility and to also include eligibility for immigrant children.
- Further adjust Medicare area wage indexes to reward areas with low or falling food insecurity and low rates of excess food cost burden of greater than 25 percent of income.
- Instate a special tax on high-cost restaurant meals (more than $40 per person) in areas with high or rising food insecurity, with proceeds going to local food banks or farmers delivering fresh produce or lean proteins to grocery stores that serve high food insecurity clientele.
- Apply a special tax deduction to incentivize donations to local food banks.
- Provide tax breaks or direct subsidies to farmers growing fresh produce or lean proteins to grocery stores that serve clientele in high food insecurity areas.
- Further provide state individual and business income tax breaks for communities that reduce or sustain low levels of food insecurity.
- Expand federal grants to support counties and local communities that address food insecurity in meaningful and measurable ways. These grants would effectively serve as prizes to those that achieve zero or near zero or substantial reductions in food insecurity.
- Reward federal and state subsidies to school districts that identify and reduce food insecurity among children and their families.
- Allow health insurers to count food support as part of their medical loss ratio.

STATE AND LOCAL GOVERNMENT ALIGNMENT

With the incentives and penalties in place at the federal level, state and local government leaders would likely begin to experience pressure from individual taxpayers, business owners, and Medicare and Medicaid providers. This pressure would likely lead them to conform to state and local policies aligned with federal housing priorities. Local governments and neighborhood food councils could then begin to take ownership of food insecurity goals.

For example, local governments could:

- Create Offices of Food Security that would have the mandate of completely eradicating food insecurity. These offices would make publicly available dashboards charting progress and coordinate collaborations with local community organizations and businesses.
- Create neighborhood councils for food security that help educate policy makers about local needs and local situations.
- Ensure coordination among economic empowerment offices, mental and behavioral health providers, schools, employers, and food access mechanisms to tailor solutions for the families with the greatest need.
- Dedicate local tax revenue to reducing food insecurity by supplementing federal food programs (e.g., increasing SNAP allotments, extending support to immigrant children, and contributing to local food banks).
- Remove regulatory barriers and increase financial incentives (tax or subsidies) to low-cost farmers markets in areas with high food insecurity.

CREATING AND PAYING FOR SUSTAINABLE SOLUTIONS

Federal and state tax policies can be applied to incentivize the desired end state of universal food security. One approach might be to identify all likely downstream beneficiaries of better food security (e.g., health organizations, schools, employers, local government units such as law enforcement and family services, local philanthropies, food producers, grocery stores, restaurants) and attempt to quantify the value of achieving universal food security for the community as a whole and where possible, for beneficiaries experiencing or at risk of food insecurity. This approach would allow for the prioritization of state and federal subsidies to address food insecurity. If more local funds are necessary to achieve universal food security, then voluntary or regulatory payment approaches could be developed that are proportional to local beneficiaries' benefits (this could be via Social Impact Bond mechanisms or CAPGI [Collaborative Approach to Public Good Investments], or new taxes or expected contributions through philanthropy). Communities that have achieved universal food security should have lower health and social service costs over time. Successful community models should be disseminated.

OUTCOME EVALUATION AND LEARNING

Program and policy outcomes and outputs must be accurately and routinely evaluated to promote the continuous improvement of interventions and policies relative to community needs. There are currently multiple ways to measure food insecurity locally; one standard measure must be agreed on. Because poverty and structural economic conditions are highly correlated with food insecurity, progress must also be rewarded. Approaching universal food security will require broad-based investments to address the intersectional drivers impacting food insecurity, which include high health care costs, structural racism, and a lack of affordable housing (Hunger and Health, n.d.). Therefore, the comprehensiveness of local plans should be a key element of targeted federal subsidies and interventions. The good news is that substantial progress is possible, as recent research has shown (Rouse and Restrepo, 2021).

REFERENCES

Hunger and Health. n.d. *Understand Food Insecurity.* Available at: https://hungerandhealth.feedingamerica.org/understand-food-insecurity (accessed July 13, 2022).

Rouse, C., and B. Restrepo. 2021. *Federal Income Support Helps Boost Food Security Rates.* Available at: https://www.whitehouse.gov/cea/written-materials/2021/07/01/federal-income-support-helps-boost-food-security-rates (accessed July 13, 2022).